Perfect Weight Loss

Kate Santon is a freelance writer and editor who specialises in food and drink. A firm believer in healthy eating, she is the author of *Need to Know GI* and *GL Diets, Need to Know Calorie Counting,* Collins' Gem guides on *GL Diets, Cholesterol* and *Fat Burning Diets,* as well as *Perfect Calorie Counting.*

Other titles in the *Perfect* series

Perfect Answers to Interview Questions – Max Eggert
Perfect Babies' Names – Rosalind Fergusson
Perfect Best Man – George Davidson
Perfect Brain Training – Philip Carter
Perfect Calorie Counting – Kate Santon
Perfect Confidence – Jan Ferguson
Perfect CV – Max Eggert
Perfect Detox – Gill Paul
Perfect Family Quiz – David Pickering
Perfect Interview – Max Eggert
Perfect Letters and Emails for all Occasions – George Davidson
Perfect Memory Training – Fiona McPherson
Perfect Numerical and Logical Test Results – Joanna Moutafi and Marianna Moutafi
Perfect Numerical Test Results – Joanna Moutafi and Ian Newcombe
Perfect Party Games – Stephen Curtis
Perfect Personality Profiles – Helen Baron
Perfect Persuasion – Richard Storey
Perfect Positive Thinking – Lynn Williams
Perfect Presentations – Andrew Leigh and Michael Maynard
Perfect Psychometric Test Results – Joanna Moutafi and Ian Newcombe
Perfect Pub Quiz – David Pickering
Perfect Punctuation – Stephen Curtis
Perfect Readings for Weddings – Jonathan Law
Perfect Relaxation – Elaine van der Zeil
Perfect Speeches for All Occasions - Matt Shinn
Perfect Wedding Planning – Cherry Chappell
Perfect Wedding Speeches and Toasts – George Davidson
Perfect Written English – Chris West

Perfect
Weight Loss

Kate Santon

BOOKS

Published by Random House Books 2009

10 9 8 7 6 5 4 3 2 1

First published in Great Britain in 2009 by
Random House Books
Random House, 20 Vauxhall Bridge Road,
London SW1V 2SA

www.rbooks.co.uk

Addresses for companies within The Random House Group
Limited can be found at: www.randomhouse.co.uk/offices.htm

The Random House Group Limited Reg. No. 954009

A CIP catalogue record for this book
is available from the British Library

ISBN 9781847945501

The Random House Group makes every effort to ensure that the
papers used in its books are made from trees that have been legally
sourced from well-managed and credibly certified forests. Our
paper procurement policy can be found at
www.randomhouse.co.uk/paper.htm

Typeset by Delineate for Grapevine Publishing Services Ltd,
London

Printed in the UK by CPI Bookmarque, Croydon, CR0 4TD

Contents

Introduction

There is good news for anybody who wants to lose weight and stay at a new, healthier level in the long term. It's perfectly possible.

However, it often seems as though the odds are stacked against success. Most of us want, at some time, to lose weight. However, trying to do so can feel like a struggle, an almost-impossible quest for a diet that will actually work, which won't lead to horrible hunger pangs but will lead to a permanently lower weight. It can be confusing: there are so many possible methods, so many different diets online and in the press, clubs to join, friends to listen to … And deep inside, we all know that most of them – maybe all of them – will not work in practice.

But it can be done. You can lose excess weight, do it in a healthy way, do it sustainably – and keep to a new and more healthy weight over time. Many people have done exactly this, and will continue to do so, and you can be one of them. There's no deep, dark secret either (though sometimes it seems that way). Lots of people are happy to say there is, that only they have found it and all you need to do in order to share it is buy their helpful products.

Unfortunately there are lots of myths floating about, particularly when it comes to what you should and should not eat, but, thankfully, there is also a wealth of practical, straightforward information that can be useful and which is based on reality. You need to set yourself up to succeed, and *Perfect Weight Loss* will provide you with strategies that can help.

Slow, sustainable change is the answer, combined with a balanced and realistic approach. People who lose weight sustainably get back in touch with what their bodies need, and with how they react. It can sound a bit boring, even academic, but it is far from being so – especially when you bear in mind that it is much, much, much more likely to bring success than any number of 'eat tropical fruit and nothing else for a fortnight' flash diets and similar pieces of nonsense. When you take this route and really understand what you are doing, you are working with your body and not against it. You have to give your body time to adapt too.

We'll begin with a reality check, one that will give you a real understanding that can only help your weight-loss campaign, and which will help you distinguish the helpful from the useless. Motivation is important, so there are also some reminders of why it might be good to lose weight, how much you should think about trying to lose, and in what sort of time. Understanding what you are doing, and how you can balance things out to achieve your aim is absolutely necessary, but so is solid, practical information – and you'll find plenty of that, from realistic advice on exercise to recipes which can help you turn your diet around. As an added bonus, *Perfect Weight Loss* ends with a section full of helpful tricks and tips from people who have successfully lost their weight and kept it off, covering everything from how to resist temptation in the supermarket to hints about the best choices and strategies when you are faced with a buffet at a party.

'Sustainable' is something of a buzz word at the moment, but that doesn't alter the fact that a realistic weight-loss plan does have to be sustainable if you want it to work in the long term. If you take it easy, making little changes that can bring both real benefits and have a real impact, building them up as you go, then the odds against success can change – and swing round in your favour. You can start them moving right now.

1 Don't 'diet'

Many of us start specific diets, whether they are apparently sensible or quite evidently strange, every day – and this is where the bad news about dieting comes in.

Beginning a formal 'diet', whatever the particular plan or scheme or even organisation concerned, is unlikely to bring the longer-term permanent change that most serious dieters want to achieve. In fact, almost half of those who start a diet stop within two weeks, and it is often said that 'diets don't work' even for those who stick with them for longer. That is more than just a flippant and dismissive comment; it is an accurate statement that has been supported by proper scientific research, again and again. An astonishing 95–97 per cent of all dieters fail to keep their lost weight off in the long term. So why don't diets work, and what can be done about it if you want to lose weight?

Formal diets, as such, don't have the effect that all dieters want for several reasons. The major one is that when you are following a diet plan, you are eating abnormally. For example, the diet might feature something unusual, like a meal-replacement milkshake; it might concentrate on a particular dish or food, such as cabbage soup or grapefruit; it might forbid eating at all after 5 p.m. or it might require you to calculate certain scores for everything you eat. Even with all the will in the world, you can only do things like this for a short or limited period of time, largely because you are struggling against the way your body (and, in some cases, your mind) works.

All living things need to find and consume fuel – food – to provide the energy they require in order to function; it's a basic biological necessity. Humans are no exception, but many of the more specific diet plans around deprive our bodies of sufficient food and essential nutrients. This is obviously undesirable in health terms, but it is also problematic in other ways. Though people following these plans may lose some weight, especially at the start, they then stop 'dieting' and inevitably return to the way they ate beforehand. All their old favourite foods feature again and these are, of course, exactly the food choices which led to the increase in weight in the first place. In this situation, dieters are bound to put their lost weight back on, most likely with a little extra. Under extremely low-calorie plans it's also possible for dieters to eat so little that they become ravenously hungry all the time. They are then in danger of becoming obsessed with food, especially with 'bad' food like chocolate and cakes, and when they stop, they reward themselves for the unpleasant time they have endured … and back comes the lost weight. Either way, it seems that dieters just cannot win.

These examples aren't exceptional reactions; everybody behaves this way when they have been 'dieting'. It is simply impossible to be restrained all of the time and to go on being restrained for ever. There is very little chance that anybody who follows these kinds of diet plans will maintain any of the weight loss they might have achieved during the diet itself. The weight might come back quickly or it might come back slowly, but thorough research has shown that it will, almost certainly, come back – remember the huge percentage: 95–97 per cent. It's not a question of willpower, or a lack of it, either; it's just that keeping the weight off in these circumstances would be next to impossible. It's not the dieters who fail, though most will undoubtedly blame themselves. It's the diets. And the more bizarre and faddish the diet concerned, the more likely it is to fail.

Then there are deadlines. These can be unrealistically short, or longer and more apparently practical, but they can all have negative effects if you're not careful. The worst are the short-term plans for losing significant amounts of weight that are so popular with the media: 'drop a dress size in a month', 'lose five pounds in five days', 'have trim thighs in 28 days'. The supply is never-ending. But – and quite apart from any of the negative health consequences arising from rapid weight loss – these quick-fix diets work, when they work at all, by imposing unusual and abnormal conditions, which are often based on a low calorie intake. If you somehow manage to follow these diets and do manage to drop a size, lose those extra pounds or trim up your thighs, you then return to your normal eating habits – and, as before, surprise, surprise, back it all comes again. Any quick results are almost always extremely short-lived. There's the effect of longer deadlines, too: the 'I'm going on holiday in six months' syndrome. For perhaps a week or so you manage to follow a low-calorie diet. Then, inevitably, you lapse – but that's not important as you've still got just over five months to fit your diet in. And so on, and so on, until you're tempted into trying crazy crash diets in desperation as the suitcases come out of storage.

Yo-yo dieting ... and the consequences

And, as if all that was not enough, there's yet another reason to avoid 'dieting' as such. Those who follow set diet plans do often manage to lose some weight, usually about 5–10 per cent of their starting weight. That's in the beginning, mind. And then the pattern of weight loss stalls and stops altogether, leading to one of (generally) two reactions. The first is further dietary restriction, dropping calorie intake levels even more. This is a slippery slope which ends up with eating disorders, and it has been estimated that up to 35 per cent of dieters may slide into 'pathological' abnormal eating patterns at some time. The other reaction is simply to give up, and blame yourself for being weak. These people, the majority, then find that their lost weight creeps back on, plus a little more.

Soon they are tempted to try again, maybe following a different plan as the first one clearly didn't work, but the same pattern just repeats itself. As before, they manage to lose some of the excess, only this time slightly less weight is lost from a slightly higher starting point, and then slightly more is regained. This pattern is often called yo-yo dieting; it is particularly common in women, and the overall effect is one of a gradual increase in weight over time. It's a marked tendency when dieters have been trying to lose weight quickly, using diets which involve particularly severe calorie restriction, but it's by no means con-fined to this type of dieting. Several different factors are involved, and they all centre around the metabolism – the way the body makes and uses energy. One possibility concerns the fact that lean tissue – muscle tissue – is more easily lost than regained, and lean tissue is more meta-bolically active than fat, which is what you tend to put on instead of muscle when you regain weight. Another is that when you subject your body to repeated bursts of calorie restriction, it cannot distinguish between this being voluntary and temporary (yet again) or imposed from without, as in a famine or similar period of food scarcity. If food is short, it's better for your body to use less of it, so it reacts to conserve its resources. This is a completely natural and protective response, and is one of the reasons why the yo-yo dieting habit can be difficult to break. It's worth making the effort, though, because yo-yo dieting is destructive. Not only is it bad for your physical health – it's been asso-ciated with an increased risk of heart disease as it appears to affect the balance of 'good' and 'bad' cholesterol in the blood – but it's also bad for you psychologically. It's comparatively easy to end up in a state of poor self-esteem, even self-loathing, as you try and deal with an endless cycle of unrealistic aims and dashed hopes, and recriminations as you beat yourself up for a failure which was simply waiting to happen.

It's time to stop

Easily said – but stopping can be very difficult to do when there is so much emphasis on 'dieting' almost everywhere you look. Though everyone can recognise that some of the schemes which crop up in magazines, sometimes endorsed by celebrities, are patently peculiar and unlikely to succeed – there's even been a fast-food diet – it is hard to ignore a general, all-pervading attitude that the only way to lose weight is to follow a strictly formal diet for a set period of time. Lots of busi-nesses tell you that this is so, from the media to the food industry, and dieting is a business like any other. In fact, it's a big business. There are few reliable figures, but the size of the diet industry in the US alone has been estimated at somewhere between US$100 billion and $40 billion, with the actual figure probably lying somewhere in between. And it's not just the US, of course. For instance, it's estimated that the British spend up to £10 million a year on diet products. Now, there are some products and ideas that come from the diet industry which you can use to help you with sustainable weight loss, but do be wary of relying on diet plans and schemes to achieve it. Most of these will inevitably fail as the odds are against success – and, of course, if they did work in the long term all the diet businesses would have to cease trading.

How to succeed

So what to do about all of this, given that you do want to lose some weight, and keep it off? First, don't lose heart because it can be done, it isn't excessively complicated and small changes can make a big difference. Remember that many people have been successful, and what most of them have in common is that they didn't 'diet'. It's time to take charge and do things for yourself, valuing yourself in the process, and not rely on the diet madness which sometimes seems to be all around us.

As far as food goes, the key is really healthy eating, not fads and fancies. Don't think 'dieting' but keep it sustainable instead. That means not restricting what you eat in unrealistic, unusual or bizarre ways and, though it will most likely mean keeping an eye on quantities, it won't mean that you have to go hungry. On the contrary: you should have three regular meals and a couple of healthy snacks too. No single industry benefits from promoting healthy food, so there's less all-pervading coverage of it in the media. Governments, however, do have a vested interest in encouraging their citizens to be healthier. They worry about obesity statistics, the increasing rates of diseases that are linked to being overweight and occasional alarming facts like the increase in the quantity of statins (drugs designed to help the fight against heart disease) being prescribed for children. There is a new official emphasis on eating well, so there is now plenty of advice about healthy eating which is easily available. There are also some negative myths and stories which need to be dispelled, however. To take just four: healthy eating doesn't have to be expensive, take hours and hours of your time, involve knitting your own muesli, and scientists don't actually change their minds about what is 'healthy' all the time; the basic guidelines are straightforward and stay roughly the same.

The other thing to do is to raise your overall activity level. That doesn't mean taking up competing in iron-man triathlons immediately or charging around cities indulging in free running – there's no need to be extreme here, either. Just be more active generally. It can even be fun, (even if you think all exercise belongs to the devil), especially if you think laterally and accept that doing something you might find more enjoyable such as dancing can also count as a perfectly valid form of exercise.

In short, you can change your weight, and change it for good. In order for weight loss to be really sustainable it's not going to happen quickly and it is going to involve changes to your lifestyle. However, these changes won't be too hard to incorporate or to get used to because they should be gentle – and permanent. They should not involve doing things like eating grapefruit for a fortnight or suddenly transforming yourself into an exercise-addicted gym bunny when you've never been near a rowing machine or elliptical trainer in your life; behaving like that would be counter-productive and even dangerous.

If it's slow, it's sustainable, and you can build on it. When you look back in a year's time, you'll realise how much you can change, and change for the better.

2 Why lose weight – and how much to lose?

Everyone who decides to try and lose some weight has a whole array of reasons for doing so. These basically fall into two categories: wanting to look different, and wanting to feel or be healthier.

Appearance

Looking different is often the reason that seems to be more important, at least at first: 'I want to be able to fit into that dress for the party', 'I would like to look better on the beach', 'I used to have a six-pack and now it's disappeared'. However, those kinds of reasons are often the ones that can push potential dieters into taking up short-term, deadline-driven diet and exercise plans. That doesn't mean you should automatically decide to ignore this particular aspect of weight loss completely, of course, but do be aware that it is a rather unsustainable motivator if it is your only one. The simple desire to change your appearance can also lead to the almost unconscious assumption that if you do manage to lose a bit of weight, other problem areas in your life will also change for the better. They just might – losing weight can bring about an increase in self-confidence and that can have interesting consequences in itself – but generally lowering your weight won't make a difference to unrelated matters. Once again, it is vital to be realistic, especially as this needs to be a long-term project, a real lifestyle change.

It is worth bearing in mind that some people's reactions to a weight-loss campaign can be a little unnerving, and one that women in particular can experience is almost a form of sisterly condemnation –

that by attempting to lose weight, the dieter is somehow bowing to social pressure and trying to conform with a silly stereotype of female beauty. The clearest response to this argument is the health issue: being overweight has repeatedly been shown to have a bad effect on your health. And this, the second main group of reasons for losing weight, is likely to be a more lasting aid in the quest for permanent change.

Health

There is no doubt that being heavier than you should be is bad for you. Being overweight is just one risk factor for developing serious health problems, of course, but it is one you can do something about, like smoking. There are others which you can't change – such as your age or sex – and some which are difficult to tackle, like economic status, so it makes sense to target the ones you can do something about.

It's been estimated that being obese can shave as much as nine years off your life, maybe more, and simply being overweight can also have a bad impact on your life expectancy. If you are carrying too much weight you stand an increased risk of developing several serious medical conditions and requiring long-term treatment. This is why governments all over the world are concerned about increasing obesity, and it is also one of the reasons why the World Health Organisation has described obesity as a 'worldwide epidemic'. The various medical conditions and their contributing causes don't always receive the specific attention or publicity that you would think they might merit – there are no mandatory health warnings on fast food, potato crisps or chocolate biscuits, for instance – though most people do realise that being too heavy is not good for them. However, men, in particular, often tend to underestimate the risk. So it's time to look at the risks that being overweight poses to your health and wellbeing in more detail ... and there is even some good news at the end. It's not all gloom.

The more overweight someone is, the greater the danger they are in. Weight can dictate the chances of developing a heart condition, dying from a heart attack or having a stroke. Weighing too much can increase the likelihood of developing certain cancers, is strongly linked to developing type 2 diabetes, having arthritis and gout, developing gall-bladder disease and gallstones, and experiencing sleep apnoea and other respiratory problems. Some recent research has also linked it to developing Alzheimer's, though the exact mechanism is unclear and the two may simply share the same risk factors. Some of these potential threats may seem to be a long way off at present, but bear in mind that things are changing fast, that type 2 diabetes is now much more common than it used to be in younger people and children, and that some overweight kids even need statins to reduce their risk of having a heart attack. The UK's National Health Service estimates that about 9,000 deaths a year are directly related to obesity in England alone, and that over £1 billion is spent on treating the diseases and conditions which are linked to people weighing too much.

One thing to note is that almost everyone knows someone who is overweight, maybe even obese, and who also appears to be comparatively healthy. Don't be fooled: people often appear to be obese or overweight and healthy at 25, but are likely to get a nasty shock later, when diagnosed with a serious life-threatening condition like type 2 diabetes about 20 years further down the line. The risks are often less obvious in younger people, but that doesn't mean that they are not there; the chances are that long-term damage is being done. It's not worth taking that gamble when the issue can be addressed.

Let's look at four main health problems associated with weight. Don't panic, though; remember there's a lot that can be done about them, and that the more slowly you make changes, the more likely those changes are to be permanent.

Heart disease and stroke

Research project after research project, including the most enormous and long-running studies, have shown that weight and diet have a direct relationship to the chances of developing some form of cardiovascular disease – heart disease or stroke. Fatty deposits form in the linings of the arteries, restricting the flow of blood and putting a strain on the heart. Cardiovascular disease is very common – it causes almost 20 million deaths worldwide each year (200,000 in the UK in 2008) and is a major cause of premature death – so it makes sense to lower your risk, because you can actually do this very effectively. Many of the risk factors can be significantly reduced by making changes to your weight, diet and lifestyle: by losing or lowering any excess weight, eating healthily and taking more exercise.

Cancer

Obesity and simply being overweight are also major risk factors for developing certain types of cancer. For women, these are colon cancer, breast cancer, cervical, uterine and ovarian cancers and cancer of the gall bladder. Overweight men are more likely to develop cancers of the colon, rectum and prostate. It's not completely clear whether the risk is linked to simply being heavy, or whether it's linked to a diet which is high in fat and calories, but the two tend to go together anyway. Again, there's an improvement in risk when excess weight is lost, and regular exercise has also been shown to reduce the chances of some cancers occurring.

Diabetes

Type 2 diabetes, known as non-insulin-dependent diabetes mellitus or adult-onset diabetes (a name which is no longer as appropriate as it once was because type 2 diabetes is now occurring in increasing numbers of children), is directly linked to being overweight – in fact over 80 per cent of those with this type of diabetes are overweight. Yet again, it's something you want to avoid. Though it's widely perceived as being less severe than type 1 diabetes, there is no such thing as 'mild' diabetes and type 2 can lead to some of the same serious consequences. Diabetes is a major cause of early death, is implicated in stroke, heart and kidney disease, and can lead to blindness, but losing weight can reduce blood-sugar levels and lower the risk of developing it in the first place. Though there's no cure, you can reduce its impact on your body if you already have it: keep your blood-sugar levels as steady as possible with a healthy diet and lifestyle. What you eat is critical.

Joints – osteoarthritis and gout

Being overweight or obese puts extra pressure on your joints, which wears away at the cartilage that protects them. It particularly puts additional stress on weight-bearing joints such as the knees and hips, as well as the lower spine. Losing excess weight can not only reduce your chances of developing osteoarthritis, it can also reduce the impact on your joints if you already have it. Exercise is very important here, and can really help to reduce pain. Take advice from a physiotherapist about the type of exercise that will work best for you if you have joint problems.

Gout is a common form of arthritis; it is caused by high levels of uric acid circulating in the blood, which can be linked to metabolic syndrome, and that can be, in its turn, a precursor to type 2 diabetes. It is also much more common in people who are overweight and has been associated with 'rich' diets – yet again, the two often go together.

There's one general point which is significant, too. Being too heavy increases the risks you run if you need to undergo surgery. For some procedures, especially hip and knee replacements, patients are often asked to lose weight beforehand and to keep it off afterwards to increase the chances of success.

And the good news? Well, simply that all of this can be turned around. Losing just 5 per cent of your present body weight, and keeping it off, can have an immediate impact on your level of risk. Losing 10 per cent improves matters even further, but in both cases this has to be slow, steady weight loss; a rapid reduction in weight can cause many other problems. It's worth remembering that you don't have to be really thin in order to be healthy, and being too thin can increase rather than reduce risk, but you do have to try and avoid being overweight or obese. If you are already obese or overweight, then losing weight could improve your life expectancy.

A healthy weight for you

There's no straightforward response to the question of exactly what constitutes a healthy weight, which might seem surprising – there are so many variables involved that there's no such thing as a simple answer. One size definitely does not fit all and no single healthy weight could be made to apply to a lot of different people – even in an ideal world not all people of the same height would weigh exactly the same.

However, though a single specific ideal weight is almost entirely impossible to determine, it is possible to arrive at a *range* of ideal weights. No one method of determining that range is perfect by itself, but you can come up with a satisfactory personal range by doing a little tweaking and being realistic. It is worth spending some time on this because it is extremely useful to have some sort of framework when you are trying to lose weight: a plan for where you are heading and a sensible target. A little time spent at the start can bring rewards later and, once again, realism is the key to success. Keep your goal attainable; don't aim for the impossible.

Individuality matters, despite what some simple charts, especially height and weight charts, might imply. To take a couple of examples, genetic inheritance and racial origin can affect how much you should weigh in order to be healthy. Genetic inheritance, in particular, has been getting some publicity recently. There is some scientific evidence that there may be an inherited predisposition to being overweight or obese. If identical twins are brought up apart, they tend to be roughly the same weight despite having a different upbringing; people whose closest relatives are thin are also likely to be thin, and not just because they share the same environment. The reasons why this is so seem to be connected to metabolism – the way the human body uses energy – and is one of the explanations for why some people put on weight while others do not, even though they are eating the same food. However, genetics does not account for the general increase over the last 30 years in the number of people who are obese and overweight – that's far too short a time span for evolutionary change. Rather, the increase is thought to be due to various environmental factors, such as the easy availability of high-calorie foods and a decreasing level of everyday exercise. Genetic factors may mean that one person has to work harder than another in order to lose weight, unfortunately, but it does not mean that it's impossible. Saying 'it's my genes' is, by and large, exactly what it sounds like – an excuse.

Measurements

It is best to start anew when trying to calculate a healthy weight range, and not make any assumptions which may be long out of date. For this reason, and for ease, all the calculations in this book are in metric – in the UK or US, you are probably more likely to 'know' your weight and height in stones, pounds, feet and inches than you are in kilos or metres. Never, ever, assume but start again with accurate measurements. The first thing to do is measure your height. Most of us haven't really had our height measured for years, so it is worth rechecking, especially as it can change slightly through life and we all fall into the trap of generalising; 'I'm just under six feet' isn't accurate enough here. The easiest thing to do is to stand against a wall or door frame with no shoes on and your head held straight. Mark the level of the top of your head with something rigid like a ruler, and mark the spot with a sticky note or pencil mark. Then measure the distance to the ground in metres, using a stiff tape measure.

Next you need to weigh yourself. You may not wish to keep weighing yourself as you try to lose weight because it can be counter-productive, but you do need a starting point. So break out the bathroom scales first thing in the morning before breakfast, but after you have been to the toilet, and weigh yourself in kilos. Make sure your scales are reliable and make a note of where you put them – on a hard surface is best – as you want to copy the same conditions every time if you are one of those people who likes a regular weighing session. If your scales are used by children, who have a tendency to bounce on or off them, or by someone with an exceptional weight (maybe you have a partner who is a bodybuilder), it will probably be worth your while to buy new ones and keep them for yourself. For the same reason, the scales in gyms can often be unreliable, as they also suffer from much more wear and tear. If you are going to weigh yourself regularly, make a mental note of what you are wearing, too, so you can replicate that as well. By the way, even if you are a regular weigher, never weigh yourself more than once a week (once a fortnight is perfectly fine) as there are completely natural fluctuations in body weight which can distort your figures and which may prove discouraging. The last thing you want to do is start weighing yourself every day and changing what you eat in response.

So, make a note of both your height and weight, but you won't need them for the first and simplest assessment ...

Waist and hip measurements

One of the clearest indicators that your weight could be putting your health at risk is a very simple one – your waist measurement. It doesn't give you any guidance about how much you should be hoping to weigh in the future or how much you need to lose in order to get there, but it is useful as a general guide because the most dangerous area in which to carry excess fat is around the middle.

Fat in this area is known as mid-section fat, visceral fat, central obesity or even abdominal adiposity, and people who have too much fat around their waist and chest are often described as 'apple-shaped'. Having excess fat around your waist puts you at much greater risk of developing diabetes and heart disease, high blood pressure, high cholesterol and high levels of blood sugar than pear-shaped people who carry their extra fat around their thighs and hips. It means you are accumulating fat internally, around your vital organs, as the name 'visceral fat' indicates, and there is some suggestion that this abdominal fat can operate in a different way from fat elsewhere in the body. It's also one of the reasons why ethnic origin can be a variable risk factor; people from some racial groups, such as many who have an Asian background, just have proportionately more body fat in this region.

So no guessing, assumptions or trying to remember what your waist once measured. If you can, find the mid-point between your lowest rib and the upper part of your hip bone – for most people, this will be at about the same level as the navel though perhaps not exactly on it – and measure around your waist in centimetres with a soft tape measure. Don't draw your breath in excessively as you do so, don't pull the tape measure in uncomfortably and keep it straight, parallel with the floor.

If you are a woman, and your waist is over 80cm, then it is too large and your health is at risk. If it is over 88cm, you are considered to be at high risk. For men, the figures are 94cm for elevated risk and 102cm for high risk. The figures are slightly different for South Asian men, who are considered to be at risk at waist measurements over 90cm, though their high-risk figure remains 102cm.

Another way of assessing risk is the waist-to-hip ratio, but a simple waist measurement is just as good an indicator. Should you wish to confirm your risk level, just divide your waist measurement by your hip measurement, keeping the measurements metric. If you are a woman with a ratio above 0.85, you're at risk; for men, the equivalent is over 1.0. You should be trying to reduce the ratio by losing weight and taking more exercise.

Finally, some people find that their waistline has expanded even though they have not gained a significant amount of weight. This is particularly true of middle-aged men, who often find that they accumulate abdominal fat as they get older; here muscle bulk is being replaced by fat. An expanding waistline, even if there is no overall weight increase, is still a sign of increasing risk. If this is true of you, you should look at the whole question of diet and exercise.

So now you know if your health is at significant risk. It's time to address the question of what might be an appropriate weight and how much you should lose, assuming you need to.

Height and weight charts – and build

For many years, simple height and weight charts were used to determine how much people should weigh, and they are still used exclusively on occasion. There were other methods of judging how much fat people were carrying – like pinches of fat around the waist – but they were often misleading. Height and weight charts were also often unsophisticated and paid little attention to normal variability, so that every woman who was the same height, say 1.7 metres tall, was supposed to weigh between 60 and 65 kilos. Using these weights as targets could be problematic, because everyone is different.

Build is one of the ways in which we differ. Some people simply have a bigger build than others of the same height; it's not just a question of excess fat. If you do manage to get down to a weight which would be more appropriate for someone of a lighter build, you'll find your new weight impossible to sustain; you will probably also look 'wrong': just too thin as well as generally unhealthy. It is easy to make assumptions about build, though. In particular, beware of assuming that you have a large build because you are tall, or a slight build if you are short – it doesn't follow.

A rough and ready way of assessing your build is looking at your wrists. That's not as mad as it sounds; if you compare yourself with friends of a similar height and weight you'll see differences, and wrists don't tend to be affected by weight gain in the same way as other parts of the body. So make a circle with your thumb and forefinger around one of your wrists (and remember that most people will have one wrist bigger than the other, depending on whether they are right- or left-handed; go for the smaller of the two). If your fingers meet, you have a medium build. If they overlap a lot, you have a small build, and if they don't meet at all you have a large one. You need to bear your particular build in mind when looking at the most popular way of judging weight at present – the BMI – and setting yourself a target.

The BMI

Height and weight charts once reigned supreme; now that position has been taken by the BMI or Body Mass Index. The BMI is another measure of weight adjusted to take height into account, and is a predictor of the risk of developing those diseases related to weight. It isn't a measure of body fat as such. Like height and weight charts, it is often used in isolation, and it isn't perfect either, though it has become so ubiquitous – it's in use everywhere from doctors' surgeries to women's magazines – that you could easily assume it was the answer to everything.

The BMI does do a good job of allowing for the fact that taller people just weigh more. What it doesn't do is allow for the fact that muscle weighs more than fat (so an extremely fit ballet dancer or body-builder would appear to be unhealthily high on a BMI chart); nor does the BMI include any variation for sex or build. Similarly, if your waist size has increased but your overall weight has not, you would still be putting your health at risk, even if your BMI fell in the 'healthy' range, and the BMI may not be entirely reliable for older people who can lose lean tissue. Finally, BMI charts are not relevant for pregnant women or anyone under the age of 18 or so – there are special ones for children and young people who are still growing. Having said all that, the BMI is still useful and you can adjust your interpretation of it slightly so that it is more applicable to you on a personal level.

There are several ways of establishing your BMI, and you'll find a chart on pages 26–7. Find your height on the chart, and trace the line downwards until it intersects with one coming across from your weight: the figure at that point is your BMI.

If your precise height and weight aren't on the chart and you want a more exact figure, then you need to do some maths. Take your height in metres and square it – multiply it by itself. Next, divide your weight in kilos by the figure you got for your height squared, and that's your BMI. There are also online calculators if you don't want to get your own pocket calculator out.

BMI figures are divided into ranges:

18.5 or below: Underweight. You weigh too little to be in the best of health, and need to eat more healthy food to ensure that your body is getting the energy and nutrients it requires in order to function properly. Try eating a little more at each meal and make sure you have a few (healthy) snacks. If your BMI is below 15 you should see your doctor.

18.5–24.9: This is considered to be the best range, but you still need to ensure that your overall diet is healthy too. There has also been some concern that the top end of the band is too high for optimum health.

25–29.9: Overweight. Your health would benefit if you lost some weight and, importantly, avoided adding any more. If your reading falls into this band you should be checking your diet, watching portion sizes (you'll still put on weight eating healthy food if there's too much of it) and taking more exercise. Go for small, gentle changes and you'll get there.

30–34.9: Moderately obese, or obese (class 1). You are putting your health at significant risk – among other things, you are ten times more likely to develop type 2 diabetes than you would be otherwise – so you should act. There's no need to despair but regard this as a wake-up call instead; it's far from being too late to turn things round. Whatever you do, don't be tempted into panicking and trying crash diets, as they could just add to your level of risk. Again, set sensible targets and make those changes, because they will be of real benefit.

35–39.9: Severely obese or obese (class 2). You are quite likely to already know that you are putting your health at risk, and you really need to start doing something about it if at all possible. At these figures you should definitely talk to your doctor, partly because you could damage your health further if your weight-loss efforts are too extreme and partly because it's another level of help which can be very useful.

40 and above: This is the category known as morbidly obese, and being in this group poses a very serious risk. You should get advice from your doctor as soon as possible, and probably also from a registered dietitian (they are properly regulated in the UK and elsewhere; what you don't want is someone who promises you the moon or comes up with mad plans).

At present, it is thought that the healthiest BMI, assuming you are not a ballet dancer or bodybuilder, is about 21.0. If your BMI is over 30, then your weight is markedly increasing your risk of developing heart disease or diabetes. Even BMIs of over 25 have been shown to increase risk significantly – indeed the figures for high blood pressure show an

BMI chart

HEIGHT IN METRES

WEIGHT IN KILOGRAMS

	1.52	1.54	1.56	1.58	1.60	1.62	1.64	1.66	1.68	1.70	1.72
46	19.9	19.4	18.9	18.4	18	17.6	17.1	16.6	16.3	15.9	15.5
48	20.8	20.2	19.7	19.2	18.7	18.3	17.8	17.4	17	16.6	16.2
50	21.6	21.1	20.6	20	19.5	19.1	18.6	18.1	17.7	17.3	16.9
52	22.5	21.9	21.4	20.8	20.3	19.8	19.3	18.8	18.4	18	17.6
54	23.3	22.8	22.2	21.6	21.1	20.6	20.1	19.6	19.1	18.7	18.2
56	24.2	23.6	23	22.4	21.9	21.4	20.8	20.3	19.9	19.4	18.9
58	25.1	24.5	23.9	23.2	22.7	22.1	21.6	21	20.6	20.1	19.6
60	26	25.3	24.7	24	23.4	22.9	22.3	21.7	21.3	20.8	20.3
62	26.8	26.2	25.5	24.8	24.2	23.7	23	22.4	22	21.5	20.9
64	27.7	27	26.3	25.6	25	24.4	23.8	23.2	22.7	22.1	21.6
66	28.6	27.8	27.2	26.4	25.8	25.2	24.5	23.9	23.4	22.8	22.3
68	29.4	28.7	28	27.2	26.6	26	25.3	24.6	24.1	23.5	22.9
70	30.3	29.5	28.8	28	27.3	26.7	26	25.4	24.8	24.2	23.6
72	31.2	30.4	29.6	28.8	28.1	27.5	26.8	26.1	25.5	24.9	24.3
74	32	31.2	30.4	29.6	28.9	28.2	27.5	26.8	26.2	25.6	25
76	32.9	32	31.3	30.4	29.7	29	28.2	27.5	27	26.3	25.7
78	33.8	32.9	32.1	31.2	30.5	29.8	29	28.3	27.7	27	26.4
80	34.6	33.8	32.9	32	31.2	30.5	29.7	29	28.4	27.7	27
82	35.5	34.6	33.7	32.8	32	31.3	30.5	29.7	29.1	28.4	27.7
84	36.3	35.4	34.6	33.6	32.8	32.1	31.2	30.4	29.8	29.1	28.4
86	37.2	36.3	35.4	34.4	33.6	32.8	32	31.1	30.5	29.8	29.1
88	38.1	37.2	36.2	35.2	34.4	33.6	32.8	31.9	31.2	30.4	29.7
90	39	38	37	36	35.1	34.3	33.5	32.6	31.9	31.1	30.4
92	39.9	38.8	37.9	36.8	35.9	35.1	34.2	33.3	32.6	31.8	31.1
94	40.7	39.7	38.7	37.6	36.7	35.9	34.9	34	33.3	32.5	31.8
96	41.5	40.5	39.5	38.4	37.5	36.6	35.7	34.8	34	33.2	32.4
98	42.4	41.3	40.3	39.2	38.3	37.4	36.4	35.5	34.7	33.9	33.1
100	43.3	42.2	41.1	40	39.1	38.2	37.2	36.2	35.5	34.6	33.8
102	44.1	43	42	40.8	39.8	38.9	37.9	37	36.2	35.3	34.5
104	45	43.9	42.8	41.6	40.6	39.7	38.7	37.7	36.9	36	35.1
106	45.9	44.7	43.6	42.4	41.4	40.4	39.4	38.4	37.6	36.7	35.8
108	46.7	45.5	44.4	43.2	42.2	41.2	40.1	39.1	38.3	37.4	36.5
110	47.6	46.4	45.3	44	43	42	40.9	39.9	39	38.1	37.2

HEIGHT IN METRES

		1.74	1.76	1.78	1.80	1.82	1.84	1.86	1.88	1.90	1.92	1.94
	46	15.1	14.8	14.5	14.2	13.9	13.5	13.3	13	12.7	12.5	12.2
	48	15.8	15.5	15.1	14.8	14.5	14.1	13.8	13.6	13.3	13	12.7
	50	16.5	16.1	15.8	15.4	15.1	14.7	14.4	14.1	13.8	13.5	13.3
	52	17.1	16.8	16.4	16	15.7	15.3	15	14.7	14.4	14.1	13.8
	54	17.8	17.4	17	16.6	16.3	15.9	15.6	15.3	14.9	14.6	14.4
	56	18.5	18.1	17.7	17.3	16.9	16.5	16.2	15.9	15.5	15.1	14.9
	58	19.1	18.7	18.3	17.9	17.5	17.1	16.7	16.4	16.1	15.7	15.4
	60	19.8	19.4	18.9	18.5	18.1	17.7	17.3	17	16.6	16.3	16
	62	20.5	20	19.5	19.1	18.7	18.3	17.9	17.5	17.1	16.8	16.5
	64	21.1	20.6	20.2	19.7	19.3	18.9	18.5	18.1	17.7	17.3	17
	66	21.8	21.3	20.8	20.4	19.9	19.4	19.1	18.7	18.3	17.9	17.5
	68	22.4	21.9	21.4	21	20.5	20	19.7	19.2	18.8	18.4	18.1
	70	23.1	22.6	22.1	21.6	21.1	20.6	20.2	19.8	19.4	19	18.6
	72	23.8	23.2	22.7	22.2	21.7	21.2	20.8	20.4	19.9	19.5	19.1
	74	24.4	23.9	23.3	22.8	22.3	21.8	21.4	21	20.5	20	19.7
	76	25.1	24.5	24	23.4	23	22.4	22	21.5	21	20.6	20.2
	78	25.7	25.1	24.6	24	23.6	23	22.5	22.1	21.6	21.2	20.7
	80	26.4	25.8	25.2	24.7	24.2	23.6	23.1	22.7	22.1	21.7	21.3
	82	27.1	26.4	25.9	25.3	24.8	24.2	23.7	23.2	22.7	22.2	21.8
	84	27.7	27.1	26.5	25.9	25.4	24.8	24.3	23.8	23.2	22.8	22.3
	86	28.4	27.7	27.1	26.5	26	25.3	24.8	24.4	23.8	23.3	22.9
	88	29	28.4	27.8	27.1	26.6	25.9	25.4	24.9	24.4	23.8	23.4
	90	29.7	29	28.4	27.8	27.2	26.5	26	25.5	24.9	24.4	23.9
	92	30.4	29.7	29	28.4	27.8	27.1	26.6	26.1	25.5	24.9	24.5
	94	31	30.3	29.6	29	28.4	27.7	27.2	26.6	26	25.5	25
	96	31.7	31	30.3	29.6	29	28.3	27.7	27.2	26.6	26	25.5
	98	32.3	31.6	30.9	30.2	29.6	28.9	28.3	27.8	27.1	26.5	26
	100	33	32.2	31.5	30.9	30.2	29.5	28.9	28.3	27.7	27.1	26.6
	102	33.7	32.9	32.2	31.5	30.8	30.1	29.5	28.9	28.2	27.6	27.1
	104	34.3	33.5	32.8	32.1	31.4	30.7	30	29.5	28.8	28.2	27.6
	106	35	34.2	33.4	32.7	32	31.2	30.6	30	29.4	28.7	28.2
	108	35.6	34.9	34	33.3	32.6	31.8	31.2	30.6	29.9	29.3	28.7
	110	36.3	35.5	34.7	34	33.2	32.4	31.8	31.2	30.5	29.8	29.3

WEIGHT IN KILOGRAMS

increase at BMIs of over 22. There is some indication, though, that the value of the BMI as a predictor of risk is linked to age. People who are younger have much better health if they have a lower BMI; for those over 70, it's not so important. There is also the question of how long, for instance, an individual may have been obese or severely underweight.

For greater personal relevance, you can add into the basic BMI some rough consideration of your particular build and sex. Men, generally, should be at the top end of each range because they have a greater proportion of muscle mass, and women – generally again – at the lower end, because of the relative proportions of body fat to muscle. Women with small builds (remember the wrist test above), would ideally be nearer the lower end of a band than those of a larger build.

None the less, and as a sweeping generalisation, but one which is supported scientifically, most people with a BMI of 25 or more would be much healthier if they reduced it, even given all the qualifications about the BMI's shortcomings.

Combining methods – and finding a range for you

Right, now you know if you are at risk (you have measured your waist), what your build really is (roughly – you have checked using your wrist) and what your BMI is. And you aren't a ballet dancer or a bodybuilder. So how do you tie these figures together and work out a realistic weight loss target?

The easiest way to demonstrate this is to look at a fictional example: Sam. She is a woman in her thirties who recognises that she's overweight. She is comparatively short at 1.60 metres, and weighs 74 kilos; however, she's quite curvy and has a waist measurement of 80cm, so she knows she's at borderline risk as far as that is concerned. She certainly doesn't want to increase this level of risk, and would preferably like to reduce it. Checking her build, she discovers that her fingers just meet around her wrist; she's got a medium frame.

Now for her BMI. As she is, the BMI chart gives her a BMI of 28.9 – certainly in the overweight band and getting quite close to obese. Bearing in mind that she wants to move into the healthy band of between 18.5 and 24.9, she checks the chart again. She finds the position on the column for her height where those figures appear – and discovers that she would need to weigh between 48 and 62 kilos. She's female, so she should be looking at the lower end of the band, but she's got a medium build, so perhaps not right at the bottom … In an ideal world she thinks her BMI would be between 21 and 22, and that would mean her weighing about 54–56 kilos. That looks all right.

But it also means that she would have to lose a huge amount, almost 20 kilos, to get there. When faced with a figure like that it is easy to have one of two extreme reactions. The first is for her to assume it's impossible and walk away laughing. The second is to find the most freaky crash diet she can and starve herself. There's no need to fall into either trap. This is where reality needs to kick in for Sam and anyone else in a similar position, together with the remembrance of the fact that even losing 5 per cent of current body weight can bring health benefits.

SMART goals

There was, and sometimes still is, a fashion in business for referring to ideal goals as being SMART. There are various interpretations of the acronym, some of which seem repetitious, but among the most popular are Specific, Measurable, Attainable, Realistic and Time-based (or Trackable). The idea is that success will be more likely if you get all of these factors right. Weight-loss goals can certainly be all of these, and perhaps the most important are the last three, the ART.

Sam has her specific goal in mind, but she recognises that it is ambitious, to say the least. Reaching it would mean losing a large percentage of her current body weight, even though she has allowed for her medium build and avoided the very lowest end of the band. Instead she decides to keep her goal in mind, but to set a more attainable and realistic goal of 10 per cent of her body weight – and losing 7.5 kilos. That would take her to 66.5 kilos, and at 66 kilos her BMI would be 25.8, at the bottom of the overweight band but very close indeed to the boundary between that and the 'healthy' band. That would be an attainable and realistic goal, for the present.

Now for the time that would take. Sam knows that for weight loss to be sustainable (an alternative to 'specific' in the SMART acronym), she needs to lose weight slowly. She's willing to do that, knowing how stupid crash diets can be and how likely swift weight loss is to tip dieters into a pattern of yo-yo dieting, so she sets herself the aim of losing half a kilo a week, or even half a kilo a fortnight – she doesn't mind that, as long as the overall trend is downwards. She also recognises that there will be some weeks where losing weight will be almost impossible, such as Christmas. But she doesn't object to the slow pace; once her extra weight has gone, she wants it to stay away. Deadlines can be dangerous when it comes to weight loss, but a general 'slow and steady' picture can be helpful, so Sam decides to set herself a rough time of 20 to 24 weeks for this first stage. It seems long, but the more gradual the weight loss, the less likely that the extra weight will return.

Once Sam gets to her 66.5 kilos – and she does, following a sensible pattern – she stops and tries to keep her weight steady for a while, just maintaining the new weight for 12 weeks or so. This gives her body a chance to adapt to its new weight. Then, having stayed at about 66–67 kilos for three months, she tries to lose a further 5 per cent. That takes her down to just over 63 kilos – and there she is, inside the healthy band of the BMI. Another pause, keeping the weight steady, and another 5 per cent drop. Now she's on 60 kilos, and has a BMI of 23.4. That's not quite where she wanted to be at the start, but she also knows that she's doing a lot more exercise and has built muscle, so she's quite happy with this figure. Because her weight loss has been slow and steady, and because her goal was realistic rather than wildly overambitious, her new weight is sustainable rather than temporary. She has also changed her lifestyle in the process, almost without realising it.

Run the same process for your own measurements and see how it works out for you. Then check your goals and make sure they really are attainable and realistic, with no wishful thinking or assuming that nothing will change when you're on holiday. And keep it slow: don't, whatever you do, try and lose more than half a kilo a week; that really would be unsustainable. You don't have to set yourself a time if you don't want to, but do make sure your goal is trackable if you don't –

either be prepared to weigh yourself regularly, or find a garment that's tight on you at the moment and judge your weight loss by the way the fit alters as you go.

Now let's look at how all of this is going to happen in practice.

3 Making it happen

One of the most important things you can do when you are trying to lose weight is to make sure you know what you're doing. If you are informed, then it acts in your favour. Stupid myths, hype, scare stories, uncertainties and nonsense won't affect you, and you'll see clearly what you are doing and understand why you are doing it. If you can also hang on to a balanced and gradual approach, you'll make the right choices almost instinctively in time, and get to where you want to be. You already know where that is in terms of a realistic estimate of weight to be lost and the time you would like it to take.

Starting out - the food diary

Information is key, and the first piece of information which can help comes from what you are eating right now, before you start changing your diet. Keep an accurate food diary for a whole week, and do so on an ordinary week – not one where you're on holiday or doing something else unusual. List, day by day, what you eat and when you eat it, but don't make any changes. Be as specific as possible. This is difficult (it can be embarrassing to write down exactly how many packets of crisps got eaten when you were out with the gang) but there's a tendency for the act of observing something to inspire a change, so do try to be honest with yourself. If you normally have a Chinese takeaway on a Friday night, don't suddenly replace it with salad; have your takeaway and write down a specific description of it, not just a blanket term like 'Chinese' (something along the lines of 'sweet and sour pork, beef in black bean sauce, one portion of egg fried rice'). If you find yourself standing in a kebab shop at midnight, buy what you would normally buy – but write it down, even if you do so later.

Some things will be easier than others to list, as they come in convenient-to-describe portions, such as 'four fish fingers' or 'a small tin of baked beans'. For the rest, don't bother weighing or measuring; just note how much of your plate something covers – for example, 'half a plate of chips' or 'a bowl of tomato soup'. If you're cooking, jot down how you cook; whether your bacon is fried or grilled, for instance. Note the time of day by each item, and try not to omit anything. Be particularly careful of things which you barely notice – the cappuccino and biscotti on the way to work, the mid-afternoon biscuits, the things which the children haven't quite finished but which you polish off. If anything strikes you about *why* you are eating what you are eating, write it down; perhaps you eat the kids' leftovers because it would be wasteful to throw them away, or you suddenly realise that your chocolate bar on the train home has become a habit. Note milk and sugar in tea or coffee, and don't forget alcohol either. It seems tedious, but keeping a food diary like this is a great way to pinpoint those things which may be easy to change as well as the things which could be more problematic. It also helps to highlight any sneaky little habits which might undermine your weight-loss efforts. It is important, though, to be honest with yourself, and to keep it up for a full seven days. Add another day if you missed one; you need to get a picture of the whole week. It is also a good habit to get into, as keeping a record can help, particularly if things begin to drift a bit.

Try not to look at the diary as a whole until the week is over, then read it through when you've got some time to think about it. You might be horrified. Did you really eat all that chocolate, drink that much beer? Surely you didn't really have that many slices of bread in one day?

Don't act on this information just yet, though. It is important that you don't try and change everything at once; you might manage it for a few days, but that would be all. Anyway, why should you suddenly start punishing yourself? (That's what it feels like if you do.) Completely sustainable, remember? You just need to make your new, healthier approach suit your life – and in order to do that, you need to know your flash points and be fairly objective about your weaknesses when it comes to food and drink. So take a more measured look at your diary. It can be helpful to take an overview, either looking at particular times of day, at whether there's a different pattern at the weekend, or even at listing how much of particular things like bread or chocolate or vegetables or milk you ate and drank over the week as a whole. If you do that you'll probably notice that something stands out, like very little fresh fruit or a vast amount of toast. Patterns will become clearer too; an almost-unnoticed tendency to have a glass of wine when you get in from work, to nibble biscuits in a meeting or polish off peanuts in a bar. Every weekday might see you popping into a coffee shop on your walk to the office and buying a chocolate bar on your way home; or sitting down with a croissant after you've taken the kids to school. You may not have quite realised just how often you and your colleagues went to a bar at lunchtime, or how much you ate during the day even though you didn't find time to sit at the table and have a proper meal.

Next, look at some of the possible reasons why you ate what you did. These may be things you wrote down at the time, or they may be thoughts which strike you as you look at your diary. Maybe, when it comes down to it, you only have that Friday-night takeaway because your partner likes it – and you might discover that they're only having it because they think *you* like it. If you can't think of a reason, other than convenience, for why you always stop and get a large frothy coffee and a croissant, ask yourself: do you really need to do it? Could you change to a black Americano, perhaps, and have a healthier breakfast at home? Or start by just changing the coffee? (That, by the way, would be nearly 200 calories less than your cappuccino, and maybe more depending on which coffee shop you go to and how big your drink is.) Perhaps the children are leaving food because they are overfed; could you serve them a bit less? Maybe you still love your post-pub kebab, but you could cut it down to one a fortnight by simply not crowding into the kebab shop with the others. Now you are beginning to see where changes could come in, and how you could implement them.

Habits

Some researchers have said that it can take as little as three weeks to break a habit and that may be so, but it can also be much more difficult. Still, old habits don't have to die hard. Often the habits we have with what we eat and drink are connected to other habits – like pleasing a partner by agreeing to the Friday takeaway, for instance. It's worth examining these, but do be careful that you aren't tempted to procrastinate and put changes off. Often the most difficult habit for us to break is the one where we think about doing something rather than actually doing it. So do it.

If your habit is one you are particularly attached to, but which is also particularly bad (smoking is an obvious example, but from the dieting point of view so is having six packets of crisps in the pub), then it may be worth stopping altogether rather than trying to wean yourself off it gradually. If you need to, think of yourself as an addict, a crispaholic. No crisps at all may be the key, since moderation is almost impossible for you in some circumstances, particularly when alcohol is also involved.

Don't skip the science bit

Another element of information that can help when you are making decisions about food and exercise is the basic science behind weight loss. The overall picture is a complex web of interactions, but you don't need to understand the full details of every phase in every action when you're trying to lose weight; knowing the basics can help you make wise choices, and it can also help you recognise nonsense for what it is.

Calories

Everyone has heard of calories, but not everyone realises exactly what a calorie is. It's just a measure of energy and is most often used to measure the energy value of food, the amount of energy a particular food makes available to the body when it is broken down. The term 'calorie' has generally come to be used as a synonym for kilocalorie, although, scientifically speaking, a calorie is a thousandth of a kilocalorie. Calories are not a measure of fat; all food and drink except plain water has a calorie value of some kind, regardless of what it is. So you could eat 1,000 calories in cabbage, crisps or crab cakes and the amount of energy your body received would be exactly the same even though the quantities (in weight) would be different. The most significant difference comes in the nutritional benefit or otherwise of what you have consumed.

Your body will use the energy that it needs in order to function, and then it stores the rest. And that is where the problem comes in. If you consume more energy than your body uses, it hangs on to it in the form of fat. Ostensibly, this looks straightforward; just balance what you eat with what your body uses, and you should stay at a steady weight. But it's not quite as simple as that. There are lots of factors that come into play, ranging from the particular – some bodies just seem to store excess energy as fat more easily than others – to the more universal, like the role that hormones can play.

Insulin

Again, almost everyone has heard of insulin, and probably most often in association with diabetes. But this hormone, which is secreted by the pancreas, has a vital role for all of us, not just for diabetics, and can be important when we are trying to lose weight. To understand how, you need to understand a little of what happens during digestion with particular attention to glucose (sugar).

When we eat food, it is broken down by the body into molecules which can be absorbed and used for energy. Enzymes are secreted in the digestive tract which do this, and most digestion happens in the small intestine. Some things, starches, 'simple' carbohydrates (and alcohol), are broken down in the stomach first. One of the most significant products of this is glucose, the primary fuel for the cells of the body. Its simple sugar molecules are then absorbed into the bloodstream rapidly, where they cause a sharp rise in blood-sugar levels. This rapid rise is followed by an equally rapid plunge downwards, and by signals telling the body to boost glucose levels again by eating something. Everyone has experienced this effect – we've all felt hungry, grabbed a bar of chocolate or some sweets, felt hungry again soon afterwards and eaten some more. The boost of energy we get from these calorie-dense, high-sugar foods is short lived, and the resulting drop in blood-sugar levels can make us feel hungrier than we did in the first place.

The hike in blood sugar is followed by an equal rise in insulin, which helps glucose molecules enter the body's cells so they can be used for energy (insulin is also linked with fat storage). The cells take up the glucose, the level circulating in the blood drops away, and then the level of insulin falls. In reality, this is a complex balancing mechanism, but that's the essence of it. And insulin doesn't just make it possible for glucose to enter the cells of the body, it also inhibits the conversion of stored fat back into glucose which the body can use as energy.

An understanding of the way insulin works can help you to reduce hunger pangs when you're trying to lose weight. If you eat food which is digested slowly, rather than simple carbs such as white bread and sugary puddings, then you won't feel as hungry, nor will you feel hungry as quickly. Complex carbohydrates, such as those you get from vegetables, whole grains and pulses, take longer to be broken down and converted into glucose, so your blood sugar levels will be much steadier, and so will your insulin levels. Eating foods like these, which contain plenty of fibre, will slow your body's response to glucose. In short, you'll feel full for longer, and the dramatic peaks and troughs of a diet which was high in sugars and starches will become much smoother. Foods like this have a low glycaemic index figure, or GI. The GI is actually a numerical system indicating how quickly a particular type of food will cause a rise in blood sugar. Low GI foods break down slowly, and those are the ones which can make a difference in your attempt to lose weight. High GI foods, like white bread, easy-cook rice or cornflakes, are metabolised much more quickly, sending blood-sugar levels (and insulin levels, too) soaring upwards. Eating more low GI foods and fewer high GI ones isn't just good for your weight-loss effort; it's also very good for your general health.

And it's also important that you eat regularly – that helps keep blood sugar levels steady, too.

Many people – an increasing number – develop a resistance to insulin, which means that glucose is circulating in the blood for longer (excess fat around the waist seems to have a role here). As a result more insulin is produced by the pancreas to try and force a response from the body's cells, and this level of overwork can have permanent effects. Eventually the pancreas may stop producing insulin – and there you are, with type 2 diabetes, as well as many other problems. But before that stage, there will be too much insulin circulating, and someone with that happening is likely to gain weight, because of the fact that insulin also helps the body to accumulate fat in the first place.

Using energy

Now for the other side of the energy equation. Eating and drinking provide your body with the energy it needs, its input; the way it uses this energy is its output. There are essentially three elements to this: the BMR or basal metabolic rate, the thermic effect of exercise and the thermic effect of food.

The most important of these is the first one, the BMR, and it accounts for around 65–75 per cent of your energy expenditure on average – the calories your body uses. It is the basic energy the body needs in order to stay alive, because energy is used continuously, not just when you are exercising or moving about. It takes energy to pump blood around the circulatory system and keep your heart beating, to send information to the brain and receive instructions from it, to regulate your temperature, your digestion, your breathing, everything … As a result, your body is using energy even when you are asleep or resting, so it's not surprising that the BMR is so significant. The lower your BMR, the greater the risk of you gaining weight and finding it difficult to shift; the higher it is, the less likely you are to pile on the pounds.

BMR varies enormously from person to person. There's a genetic aspect to this, which is one of the reasons why identical twins raised separately and under differing conditions are likely to have a similar body weight – they have similar BMRs – but there are other variations too. Children and young people have a high BMR as they are growing, and growing bodies need more energy. Men have a higher BMR than women because they generally have more muscle mass, which uses more energy than fat. And overweight people have a higher BMR than those who weigh less – that's right, the 'slow metabolism' thing is just a myth – because it takes more energy to keep a bigger body ticking over. There are even more variations, as your body can require more energy for specific reasons, such as breastfeeding or recovering from illness, injury or surgery. A woman's BMR can fluctuate during the menstrual cycle, and the menopause can affect it as well, one of the reasons why it can be hard (but not impossible!) to lose weight after about the age of 50 or so. Nor is your BMR set for shorter periods of time; it can be affected by the action of certain hormones, such as adrenaline which is secreted if you are frightened or excited in order to boost your metabolic rate and prepare you for action. And some things you take in also have an impact, such as caffeine. This is not a licence to try and lose weight by drinking vast amounts of coffee and eating huge quantities of fine chocolate, however, as hormone levels which are raised on a regular basis are not good for you or your body.

One thing to remember here, as you lose weight, is the fact that because larger bodies have a higher BMR, your BMR will inevitably drop as the excess weight comes off. This is something you do need to consider, and is another of the reasons why slow is best – your metabolism needs time to adapt, and so do you.

The next most significant way in which your body uses energy is exercise. 'Exercise' doesn't just mean hitting the tennis court or the swimming pool in this context; it means everything you do when you are not at rest. If you fidget when watching television, that counts (but not a lot); so does brushing your hair, walking to the bus stop or doing the ironing. Exercise is a very variable part of the energy-out half of the equation; in some people it might represent as little as 10 per cent of their overall energy expenditure, while it might be as much as 50 per cent for athletes. And judging how many calories are used in undertaking any given activity is also difficult – despite tables and charts which seem to show this – because energy expenditure varies, particularly according to sex and body weight.

Exercise boosts your BMR by increasing the proportion of lean tissue (that's muscle), which burns more calories than fat tissue, so taking more exercise is one of the most important ways in which you can mitigate the negative effects of a falling BMR as you lose weight. There's also some evidence that doing more exercise is linked to improved blood-sugar and insulin levels, and to maintaining these over a longer period of time, as it can have a particular impact on mid-section fat. Exercise has been shown to reduce depression, help prevent arthritis from developing (and reduce the pain if it's already present), and strengthen bones (stronger bones, with greater bone density, mean fewer fractures). Exercise also reduces stress (don't let the exercise itself stress you out, of course) and can reduce feelings of tiredness and help you sleep more deeply when you do go to bed.

Exercise really is good for you, even if it's been somewhat overstated as a means of simply losing weight, so don't be put off if you were one of the many who found sports lessons a torture when you were at school; you don't have to play team games. In fact, you don't have to do something you might think of as a 'sport' in order to get more exercise. Check out the myths below, and find more information about specific kinds of exercise in Chapter 8.

The final way in which your body uses energy is known as the 'thermic effect of food'. It means that whenever you eat something, your body uses energy to digest it and store the resulting energy. It's a minor part of the whole – estimated at about 10 per cent at the most – and you can afford to ignore it. All it means is that if you ate a bowl of porridge which contained 150 calories, your body would use 15 of those to process your breakfast.

Myths, madness – and grains of truth

When you embark on a weight-loss programme, you suddenly notice that dieting stories really are everywhere. Magazines are packed with 'helpful' hints and tips; TV programmes tell you to eat nothing but wheatgrass or exercise like a maniac; friends and family come up with suggestions and pronouncements about what you ought to do or about what worked for a friend of a friend. Sometimes these ideas are great; sometimes – more often, unfortunately – they are either only partially useful or complete codswallop. Time for a quick look at some of the most persistent ones.

Myth: exercise is a substitute for dieting

This is a belief which is held by many people, especially men. And it's not true. It's quite clear that you would need to do a truly enormous and impractical amount of exercise to negate the effects of a poor diet. But, in actual fact, science cannot prove conclusively that exercise keeps fat at bay at all – in fact, all a recent report could conclude was that 'data to support this hypothesis is not particularly compelling' – which may seem surprising given that this idea has become received wisdom. Don't forget that exercise can make you hungry, which is probably where it falls down as a method of weight loss. If you burn more calories, you are likely to consume more as well; your body needs to make up for the energy which has been used. Most of us have also experienced the 'I've been to the gym, therefore I can have chips' justification syndrome. But this isn't a couch-potato's charter. What is clear is that lean people are more physically active, and exercise does have other important overall health benefits.

Myth: exercise has to be macho to work

Wrong – it doesn't, at all, and macho exercise is also likely to lead to injuries. It can even be dangerous if you haven't done much exercise in the past, putting a real strain on your cardiovascular system. As you increase the body's demand for energy so intensely, you'll also need to take in lots of extra calories to compensate.

Small, gentle changes can have an immediate impact and are also less likely to result in a pressing need for more food. Try increasing your current level of exercise to 30 minutes a day, and make sure you carry on with it. Most people don't see an improvement until they've been doing that amount of daily exercise for about three months, so don't give up. Walking is one of the easiest things to incorporate into your routine, and you don't have to start by storming up Snowdon. Keep your exercise a routine, not a one-off event.

Myth: muscle converts into fat when you stop exercising

Muscle and fat are different substances, and one cannot 'turn into' the other. What does happen if you stop exercising, though, is that your muscles will lose tone. Many people who once exercised regularly, and who suddenly cannot do so because of an injury, notice that they gain weight as well. The problem is that they are generally eating the same amount as they were when they were exercising. It's not the muscle 'changing'; it's energy consumption being too high for their reduced energy output, so the excess is being stored as fat at the same time that they are losing muscle bulk.

Myth: taking pills can make you lose weight

Yes, some can. But they can also be dangerous. Never contemplate taking slimming pills without talking to your doctor first; certainly don't pop something you bought online without reference to anyone who knows your medical history, as it could have adverse effects. Others might be a waste of money as they'll have no effect whatsoever, and some might have the unpleasant effect of giving you violent diarrhoea. Slimming is a great area for snake-oil salesmen and if something sounds too good to be true, it usually is. The same, by the way, applies to things you sniff, smear or stick on yourself, all of which are available as well.

Prescription slimming pills are generally only given to people who fall into the upper levels of the BMI scale, or who might have other health problems which relate to their weight. Not all of these are without their problems. Sales of one, Rimonabant, have just been suspended in Europe because there was thought to be evidence that it doubled the rate of psychiatric disorders; it has also been refused approval in the US. And prescription weight-loss drugs aren't a way of escaping lifestyle change; they have to be combined with 'diet and lifestyle management'. In these circumstances they can benefit some people who are generally over 100kg – but the World Health Organisation has pointed out that weight lost while taking tablets generally returns when the tablets are stopped. That's not the effect you want.

Myth: just take supplements

If your diet is unsound and having an adverse effect on your health, you cannot correct the damage by taking supplements; nor will they help you lose weight. When it comes to health, there have been many studies showing that antioxidant supplement tablets, for instance, are almost entirely useless when compared to eating foods high in anti-oxidants; they may work in the lab but do not have the same effect in practice. You won't improve matters by taking supplements instead of changing your diet and lifestyle.

Some mineral and vitamin supplements have been publicised as influencing weight loss, notably iodine. Yes, people who are deficient in iodine may have an underactive thyroid, which can impact on their BMR, but taking an iodine supplement like seaweed tablets without actually being deficient in iodine would not be a good idea. If you think an underactive thyroid or something similar may be your problem, you should see your doctor first.

Myth: skipping meals is a great way to lose weight

It's actually best not to skip any, and even to have a couple of snacks between meals. This will keep blood-sugar levels as steady as possible, which helps, and avoiding meals has exactly the opposite effect. A lot of people miss breakfast, but many studies have shown that those who do that are often heavier, on average, than those who don't. Skipping breakfast or lunch may seem like a good idea, but often leads to a sudden outbreak of eating high-calorie foods mid-morning or halfway through the afternoon as a consequence of plummeting blood-sugar levels. Eat regularly and well – three meals a day, plus two (healthy) snacks – with no high-sugar sweets to keep you going, and you'll find that you don't feel wildly hungry, weak, dizzy or twitchy – or tempted to reach for that biscuit (or six), or the sugary sweets.

Myth: crash diets are a good way to start a more normal diet

A crash diet is one which restricts you to a very low number of calories, usually over a short period of time, and which will almost always specify exactly what you eat (and maybe when you eat it). All formal health organisations agree that they are unlikely to succeed in the long term. But are they worth trying as a form of encouragement? Well, that depends on the individual but, generally, no. You will lose weight, but most of that weight loss will be fluid and your weight will go back up quite quickly when you stop your crash diet; as such, crash diets are a disincentive. They're not sustainable and may also put you off the whole idea of trying to lose weight because they are so restrictive, will make you feel hungry and may also make you feel odd – being dizzy and faint are common complaints. They can also be another way of procrastinating – of putting off the other changes that you should be making instead. And, of course, crash diets can lead to a pattern of yo-yo dieting; you don't want to go there. Plus, crash diets seem to encourage the loss of more muscle tissue than other weight-loss options, and that's the opposite of what you want to happen. Better to accept that slow is best, right from the start.

Myth: diets that restrict particular types of food are useful

When a diet specifies cutting out whole food groups – carbohydrates were a popular target not so long ago – it can lead to nutritional deficiency and that can have all sorts of consequences. Doing this is a hallmark, in fact, of the fad diet. There are more independent approaches than following a formal restrictive diet, though: people often, for instance, decide that a quick way to lose weight would be to eliminate dairy food. Well, yes, some dairy products are high in saturated

Deciphering media stories

When you are alert to information, it's important that you are also aware of how that information has been gathered. Not all the stories about food or diets in the media are the same, so here's a quick guide to telling what's good and what's not.

- Has the study been done on people? Many have only been done on animals and while the results may be interesting, people are too different for you to make changes to our diet as a result. If it's a new diet, has it been properly researched and tested at all, let alone on people? Some diet ideas seem to have been reached theoretically without reference to the real world.

- Has the research that is being reported been done on a large and balanced number of people? Many have surprisingly small numbers of participants.

- How long did the study last? By and large, the very long and enormous health and diet studies, like the Nurses' Health Study in the US or the EPIC (European Protective Investigation of Cancer) study in Europe, provide more thorough results. But they aren't often as interesting to report on.

- Has the research been carried out by anyone who has a vested interest in the result or links to such an organisation? If so, it may not be 100 per cent reliable. A good sign of this (it may not always be obvious) is if the study endorses a particular product. Or if the result seems counter to what you know is common sense – if it shows, for instance, that crisps are a vital part of the diet or processed food is healthier than fresh ingredients.

fat and in calories – but they also contain useful vitamins and minerals, especially calcium, which is vital, and there's nothing to support the idea that cutting out skimmed milk or yoghurt will help weight loss. In fact, if you do this you may be actively hindering that weight loss, as there is evidence that increasing the level of calcium in the diet increases the breakdown of fat, and even decreases the production of fat in the first place. There may be other, less obvious, problems with restrictive diets; for instance, diets with too much fat, especially saturated fat, and too little carbohydrate (such as a previously very popular example from the US) can actually increase insulin resistance (see page 38).

These restrictive diets can also be counter-productive as they are anything but sustainable as well as unhealthy; not only does boredom set in, putting you off the whole idea, but you are making no long-term changes that will serve you well in the future.

Myth: low-fat diets work best, so cut back on fat

Fat in food doesn't necessarily make fat in the body. There's actually very little direct evidence linking those calories specifically in fat to weight gain – and even the most thorough randomised trials have been unable to provide one. Take the Women's Health Initiative, for instance. The participants in that study who ate a low-fat diet were no healthier (in terms of reduced risk of developing cancer or cardiovascular disease) after eight years of doing so than those who had been eating higher levels of fat. Nor did they weigh significantly less.

That's probably not surprising; considering that a whole variety of low-fat diets have been pushed at dieters for years, they have been remarkably unsuccessful. There are many reasons for this, but note that fat is one of the most important things that gives food its flavour. When manufacturers produce something which is low in fat they have to compensate for the resulting lack of taste by adding a substitute, usually sugar or sweeteners.

It's worth registering that not all fats are the same, as well. Unsaturated fats – mono and polyunsaturates, including the omega-3 fatty acids – actually have positive health benefits. Saturated fat and the processed trans fats are the ones to be reduced as much as possible, because consuming too much of these can damage your health (for more, see page 58).

Myth: diet schemes are great shortcuts

Well, in some cases they can be useful. But most of these plans, such as eating by numbers or following traffic light colours, suffer from a major problem, quite apart from inflexibility – no reference to portion size. So, for instance, the early versions of Glycaemic Index diets (which have been generally welcomed by the medical profession as being effective, sensible and healthy), prohibited the consumption of watermelon, deemed too high on the GI scale. The figures had been reached by assessing the same weight of different foods, and watermelon was indeed high – but actually eating the quantity that made it so high when compared to other, denser, foods would be unusual. Marmite is another example of something which can appear unhealthy at first glance, and according to the figures per 100g it is very high in salt, but most people only eat a minute quantity at any one time, maybe 5g on two slices of toast. A very recent scheme cites olives as bad, and gives fizzy drinks a rating only slightly worse than eggs (actually a nutritional powerhouse) and cheese. Sometimes the figures seem to matter more than common sense, so keep your common-sense detectors in good order when looking at these diets no matter how plausible they may seem at first. Don't forget the sustainability mantra either – do you really want to be adding things up for ever?

Myth: scientists change their minds all the time

It can sometimes seem so, often because of the way food and diet stories are reported in the media, or because there are a lot of people out there pushing their frequently eccentric ideas (and just possibly trying to sell you something en route). But the reliable, tested fundamentals don't change.

In short, these are the guidelines: eat a healthy, balanced diet; eat a varied diet; keep your diet comparatively low in fat and strong on both vegetables and fruit; have plenty of 'complex' carbohydrates like whole-grain products; and add some lean protein, especially fish, and eggs are OK too. Eat processed foods, junk and fast food as little as possible. Cook and use fresh ingredients as much as possible, and keep tabs on portion sizes.

Now it's time to look at putting all that into practice, and doing so in a way which can help you lose weight.

4 Eating healthily

All diets work – when they work – through calorie restriction, ensuring that people take in fewer calories than they use. There's no way round this, and it is the only way to actually lose weight, so you *will* need to eat, and probably drink, less; but not all diets are the same in other aspects, of course.

The trick is to make it as painless and sustainable as possible and bring about permanent change. The most important thing to do is to make sure that you eat healthily. If you are eating a reduced number of calories – and you shouldn't have to starve in order to do that if you *are* eating healthily – then you need to make sure that the calories you do consume provide all the nutrients your body needs.

There are two things which will make an enormous difference from the start, and they are fundamental to the whole concept of a healthy diet. If you are serious about losing weight and not having to go through the process again and again, then you will need to implement them. Do so gradually, though, as gentle change is most likely to stick.

First, get rid of the junk. This means fast food, but it also means processed food to a great extent, and that includes ready meals and other 'convenience' foods. However, you don't have to turn yourself into a complete food puritan and there are some processed things without which you might find life impossible (tomato ketchup, perhaps), but if you eat a lot of this sort of food and you can reduce the quantities, you're already eating in a much healthier way. The more a food is processed, the more nutrients it loses. And that applies to 'diet' or 'healthy' ready meals just as much as it does to the rest.

As an example of why this is a good idea, think about just one aspect: the size of ready-meal portions. The packaging may say 'this serves two' and that half of it contains 386 calories, but when you open the pack you frequently find it would actually serve two very small gnats. So you eat the lot, consuming 386 calories times two, and are still ravenous a couple of hours later because of all the high-GI, processed ingredients that were included in your supper. The fat, sugar and salt levels per portion are also double if you eat the lot, of course. If you made your own equivalent, you'd have more for your 386 calories, and may even have more for less than that. You would also consume less fat, sugar and salt; you wouldn't need to break out the little tubes of artificial preservatives and you'd be much more likely to be completely satisfied by your meal. The chances are that you would also have spent less money. You might have needed to spend a little more time – might – but it has to be worth it for the disproportionate level of benefits you receive.

There's something else to consider, too: the simplest way of improving your health by cutting your salt intake dramatically is to reduce the number of ready meals and the quantity of processed food you eat.

The second immediate change is therefore tied into the first. Cooking. It helps in the quest for a healthier way of life and a smaller waist more than most things you can do, but many of us seem to have lost the knack. Over the last ten years, sales of cookery books have risen by 62 per cent in the UK, yet most people seem to be cooking less – though there are promising signs of a change just beginning. Go for it, because taking charge of what you eat is only really possible if you prepare most of it yourself. You can do it much more healthily, and probably a lot better, than anyone else; you're not going to open a packet of artificial flavour enhancers and put them in a casserole, you're going to add herbs and spices instead. If you are uncertain about cooking, and many people are, then begin with straightforward things like soups and remember that this is just a start and that little changes build into bigger ones. You don't have to produce a Michelin-starred meal, just good, healthy food – and anyone can do that. If you're really unsure of your culinary skills, you might want to consider boosting your confidence by attending an evening cookery course.

The food industry constantly stresses the advantages of its processed products because they are quick and save time (and they would say that, wouldn't they? They want you to buy their processed food and ready meals rather than cook from scratch). But time really doesn't have to be much of an issue. It's easy to adapt ordinary recipes by cutting down on the quantity of high-calorie ingredients (see page 70 for some advice), and starting perhaps with some that are very quick – even if you're just beginning.

Chapter 7 has some quick and straightforward recipes to start you off, and look out for cookery books specifically designed to provide time-saving dishes – there are some excellent ones around, and you could do worse than check out those by Nigel Slater. Cook dishes that appeal to you rather than ones that just seem easy, and bear in mind that weight-loss diets with dull food are doomed to fail.

What's a balanced diet?

There are several basic food groups and, essentially, they should all form part of a healthy diet. But the large groups – carbohydrates, protein, fat – are not mutually exclusive. Apples, for instance, are mostly water (84 per cent) with a tiny bit of protein and some fat but rather more carbohydrate (11.8 per cent). Dairy products are usually assumed to be protein, but whole milk contains more carbohydrate than it does protein or fat. A rump steak doesn't have any carbohydrate (unless some is added during cooking, perhaps if it's dusted with flour), but has over 20 per cent protein and over 10 per cent fat. So even if you were to follow a diet recommending that you cut out one of the food groups, it would be next to impossible to do so in reality. And in order to be healthy, we need all of them.

We also need micronutrients, like vitamins and minerals, for example, but in much smaller quantities, and phytochemicals – literally, chemicals from plants – are also necessary micronutrients. Let's take a look at the large food groups, and at the types of food that can (loosely) be grouped under each.

Carbohydrates

Despite what some recent diets would have us believe, carbs are not evil. Like all the major food groups, they are a vital part of our diet. The glucose they provide gives the body much of its energy and they are also needed for building non-essential amino acids which are used to create proteins. Among other benefits, carbohydrates also help to lower cholesterol, process fat and build bone and cartilage as well as the tissues of the nervous system. So, they are good for you – but not all carbs are equally good for you. The trick is knowing what to choose and what to avoid.

In the previous chapter we looked at the role that blood-sugar levels and insulin can play in weight loss, at how important it is to keep the levels of both steady, and at the glycaemic index (GI) for carbohydrates. Now for the practical implications. Making the best possible choices is what all those GI diets are about, but the GI can be used to help any weight-loss programme. Low GI foods are the ones to go for, and high GI foods are the ones to restrict.

As a rough-and-ready guide, the sweeter something is, the higher its GI is likely to be. Foods which still have some fibre, as opposed to their refined and processed equivalents, have a lower GI. Potatoes, by the way, are high on most GI scales, so watch the quantities you eat as their high GI is an indication of the effect they have on your blood sugar. You can mitigate some of this by eating them in their skins or by having them with other low GI ingredients, such as lots of vegetables or a crunchy salad. But food only has a GI value if it contains carbohydrates, so you can't rely on the GI alone as a guide for what you should eat in moderation and what you should feel free to enjoy in greater amounts.

Fibre

Having more fibre in your diet has more benefits than just helping you lose weight: it can affect your cholesterol level positively and is linked with lower rates of cardiovascular disease, with a reduced chance of developing colon cancer or diabetes, and it also reduces your chances of getting piles, constipation and developing irritable bowel syndrome. It's been tied to having higher levels of 'good bacteria' in the gut too. Fibre is a carbohydrate, though it's not a nutrient as such. It is found in plants and in food derived from plants, and comes in two forms: soluble and insoluble.

Soluble fibre is broken down in water, as you'd expect, and helps delay the absorption of other carbs. Insoluble fibre absorbs water and adds bulk to food, thus helping the digestion. But if you're not used to eating lots of whole grains or food high in fibre, do increase it gradually, and drink a little more water. The 'F' in the F-Plan Diet, a fibre-based diet from the 1980s, was said to stand for something other than just fibre … and your digestive system may need time to adjust. So take it easy, but do persist, because eating more whole grains and fibre can really help.

Grains

You can avoid spikes and sudden drops in blood-sugar levels by eating whole grains and whole-grain products, which are metabolised slowly. Not only do blood-sugar and insulin levels rise and drop more smoothly than they do when you eat refined grains, they also show much less of a peak.

The energy in whole grains is released over a greater time – it takes longer for them to be broken down into sugar molecules – and the fibre they contain helps to make you feel full. Foods like this have a lower GI, so go for whole-grain versions like wholemeal bread (brown bread is usually made from white flour with caramelising agents) and pasta, and choose brown rice whenever you can. Beans and other pulses are also great sources of fibre, as well as many other nutrients, and should be included in any healthy diet.

In theory, and it's a theory that works in practice, you will not feel as hungry or be able to eat so much when you make this change. High-GI, refined grains are completely different. They have an immediate impact on blood-sugar levels, sending them spiralling up. There's another reason to reduce them too. When the bran shell is stripped away from the grain in the refining process, grains are deprived not just of their fibre, but also of protein and vital micronutrients – vitamins and minerals such as the B vitamins and iron. In some cases these even have to be added back, by law. Better to eat them whole in the first place.

Sugars

Sugar is the ultimate carbohydrate and is so swiftly absorbed that it has the highest GI score of any food in most rating schemes; it sends blood-sugar levels soaring. It's high in calories, but though other things are higher by weight, sugar's calories are 'empty' ones: it provides no other nutritional benefits whatsoever.

Cut back on the sugar you use, and do so gradually if you have a par-ticularly sweet tooth; eliminating processed food and ready meals will help as sugar is a common ingredient, even in savoury dishes. Reduce the extra sugar you add to drinks and breakfast cereals; once you have done that you could go on to cut down on any sweetened soft drinks (and check labels on *anything*, you may be surprised by what is in some apparently healthy options), and then put biscuits on the 'cutback' list. That's just an example – do whatever suits you, but do cut back. Once you have been doing so for a while, you will find that the sugary things you previously enjoyed will now seem sickly sweet and unpleasant rather than alluring. It is worth remembering, too, that sugar isn't always listed as 'sugar' on packaging. Dextrose, maltose, malto-dextrin, levulose, corn syrup, glucose and glucose syrup and invert sugar are all forms of sugar.

Evidence is beginning to emerge suggesting that, rather like fats, all sugars may not be the same. The finger of blame is being pointed at fructose (which occurs naturally in fresh fruit, fruit juices and pre-serves), and specifically at the high-fructose corn syrup (HFCS) which is used in many soft drinks and a lot of processed foods. This is a highly processed, manufactured sweetener, derived from maize. Because it contains a lot of fructose, the sugar found in fruit, there is a tendency to assume it must automatically be healthy, but this is not so. The sugars in fruit are usually about 50 per cent fructose, 50 per cent glucose, while high-fructose corn syrup can be up to 80 per cent fructose. Fresh fruit also provides a range of nutritional benefits – fibre, vitamins, minerals and other micronutrients – which HFCS does not.

Research has shown that high levels of 'free' fructose in the diet, such as those present in high-fructose corn syrup, are linked to a wide range of negative health effects including high blood cholesterol and an impaired immune system. Consuming large amounts has also been linked to 'alarming' changes in body fat and insulin sensitivity, and it's being associated with increased obesity rates. Longer-term studies are just beginning, but in the meanwhile it's worth looking out for that corn syrup on packaging and avoiding products containing it as much as possible – very easy if you cut the processed food and drink.

Vegetables and fruit

Almost all vegetables are fantastic when it comes to being low on the glycaemic index and high in nutritional benefits – even the much-maligned and high GI potato has good levels of vitamin C, for instance – but some are outstanding.

Notable among them are those with a lot of red, orange or yellow colour, an indicator of the high levels of anti-oxidants they contain; the onion family, including leeks and garlic, which are also high in powerfully protective antioxidants; and the Cruciferae – green leafy vegetables such as kale, broccoli, cauliflower, Brussels sprouts and cabbage – which contain glucosinolates, substances that help to stimulate the body's defence against cancer. Tomatoes are packed with lycopene, which has been shown to help protect the body from both heart disease and cancer. It's more effective when tomatoes are cooked (canned ones are particularly good here) and is also fat-soluble – which means that using some oil when cooking tomatoes makes more lycopene available.

In short, eat as many vegetables as you can, and eat a wide variety. The UK's Stroke Association has suggested that everyone should 'eat a rainbow' for maximum beneficial effects, and that's a handy way of reminding yourself to go for as wide a selection as you can. By doing so, you'll be getting the widest possible range of nutrients. (And don't automatically peel vegetables if you don't have to. Taking off the peel reduces fibre content and therefore raises the GI, as well as removing those nutrients which lie close to the skin.)

When it comes to fruit you should also eat the peel wherever possible – and, again, some varieties are particularly good for you. Take blueberries, for instance. They contain huge amounts of the antioxidant anthocyanin, which gives them their lovely colour. A small serving – a couple of tablespoons – provides as much antioxidant as five whole servings of carrots, broccoli, peas or apples. It's worth experimenting with some more unusual fruits as well as those you are more familiar with, but generally go for fresh or frozen rather than tinned. Tinned fruit is often in high-calorie syrup or juice – pick the latter if necessary.

Fruit juice does not pack the same nutritional punch as the whole fruit, which is one of the reasons why you can only count it as one of the 'five a day' portions of fruit and vegetables (see below), no matter how much you drink. The sugars in fruit juice have an immediate impact on blood-sugar levels, sending them soaring, so it makes sense to reduce the overall quantity if you drink a lot.

The huge range of benefits which vegetables and fruit provide is the reason behind the various campaigns urging everyone to eat at least 'five a day'. When you are eating less in order to lose weight, this is even more important. You don't have to worry too much about what a portion actually is; think in terms of one large fruit – like an apple, pear or banana – and two smaller ones, such as plums; with anything smaller, either fruit or vegetables, go by the size of your fist. You can only count one juice or smoothie, no matter how many you have; one portion of pulses or beans and one portion of dried fruit. Vegetables which have a high proportion of starch do not count at all. For most of us this means potatoes, though yam is also very high. You do not need to worry about the starch content of other root vegetables such as carrots and parsnips, however; they are fine. Variety is key, so 16 bananas wouldn't work, either.

Again, if you're not used to eating a lot of vegetables or fruit, build up slowly. Eating three a day is better than one a day, and one a day is better than none. Try to get above five if you can, as your health would really benefit if you did so. And the more fruit and vegetables you eat, the less room there is for other things …

Oils and fats

Fat is vital; it has to be included in the diet to some extent, dieting or not. It provides energy, but is also needed for many other things: so that the body can make use of the fat-soluble vitamins A, D, E and K, for instance; for keeping the body warm and protecting the skeleton; and for making hormones. Fat provides the essential fatty acids which are critical to our health and development, and which the body itself cannot manufacture – they have to come from the food we eat – and it also gives food a lot of its flavour. So don't even think about eliminating it. Keep tabs on quantities, though, as the main problem with fat is that many of us just eat too much of it, and the wrong sort at that.

Unsaturated fats

Make sure the fat you use is the best possible type – for instance, a small pat of butter contains about the same number of calories as a teaspoon of oil, but the oil, particularly if it is olive or rapeseed oil, is much better for you. The best types are the unsaturated fats – the monounsaturated and polyunsaturated ones. High levels of monounsaturated fats are found in some plant oils – olive oil is the best here, but rapeseed, groundnut and walnut oil are all high – as well as in nuts, olives and avocados. High consumption of monounsaturates has been linked to significantly lower chances of developing any form of cardiovascular disease.

There are two major types of polyunsaturated fats. Omega-3 essential fatty acids are most notably found in cold-water oily fish like salmon, herring, sardines, tuna (though canned tuna is not as good), trout and mackerel. Good vegetable sources of omega-3s are walnuts, olive and rapeseed oil, soya beans and things made from them, dark green vegetables and linseeds, as well as sesame seeds and wheatgerm. They are needed for normal brain function and help to regulate blood pressure. Omega-6 essential fatty acids are most notably found in sunflower and corn oils; they keep the immune system functioning and aid cell growth. An averagely healthy diet seems to provide enough of these, whereas positive changes are often needed to increase the omega-3 component. If you use corn oil in cooking, try changing to olive or rapeseed – you'll still have enough omega-6 coming in from everything else you eat, but will increase your omega-3 levels.

Saturated fat

The fats to restrict or avoid as much as possible are saturated fat and trans fats, which pose the worst risk to health. Saturated fat is linked to high blood-cholesterol levels, and those are linked in turn to developing cardiovascular disease, including heart attacks and stroke. Most, but not all, saturated fat is of animal origin, so foods like butter, suet, full-cream milk and some other dairy products, lard and meat (especially red meat but also the skin of poultry) are all high in saturated fat. Coconut oil is also high in saturates, though there is evidence that the saturated fat in coconut does not have the same effect as that of animal origin. Palm oil – which is included in many commercial products – is also a highly saturated fat.

Trans fats

Trans fats are the ones to cut. If you limit processed food and ready meals, watch things like commercial brands of biscuits and cakes and are careful about what you use to spread on your bread, you should be able to restrict trans fats. Small amounts of trans-fatty acid do occur naturally in meat and dairy products, but you can afford to ignore those; the vast bulk of trans fats in food comes from commercial manufacture.

Trans fats are fats which were previously liquid – vegetable oils – but which have been treated to make them semi-solid at room temperature. They are firmly associated with high cholesterol levels and an increased rate of heart disease, as well as an increased chance of developing cancer. Manufacturers are trying to remove them as much as possible but they are still present in many products, so check labels – they are often listed as 'hydrogenated' or 'partly hydrogenated' fats. Note that when they are cut, higher levels of saturates may appear instead. Fast foods are often a major source of both saturated and trans fats – another reason to give them a miss as much as you can, if not cut them completely.

You can improve matters even further by making the healthiest choices in fresh food as well, so that means going for the best options in dairy products, fish and meat – read on – and cooking in ways which do not add any unhealthy fat. Try to use monounsaturated and polyunsaturated fats as much as you can, so if you previously used lard or butter in cooking, for instance, change to olive or rapeseed oil wherever possible to reduce your intake of saturated fat. When it comes to using low-fat spreads as an alternative to butter, always check to make sure the one you choose is high in the right sort of fats – don't forget to check for those sneaky hydrogenated fats, and try olive oil or soya spreads.

Protein

Protein is everywhere in the human body, from our bones to our skin; proteins help to give structure to the body's cells and are vital for cell growth, maintenance and repair. Like carbohydrates and fats, dietary protein also serves as a source of energy. The body also makes new proteins, such as enzymes or hormones, which enable it to function. These new proteins are made from amino acids, which are made available as protein is digested, but not every protein contains all the amino acids which the body requires. There are about 20 which are needed, and nine cannot be made in the body; they have to come from food.

Foods of animal origin (eggs, meat, dairy products, fish, shellfish, and products derived from them) provide 'complete' proteins – those that contain all of the essential amino acids. Plants also provide proteins, but most are 'incomplete' proteins; they do not provide the complete range of amino acids (there are a few exceptions, such as soya beans and quinoa); to get all the essential amino acids the body needs they have to be combined with other plant sources. So if you are relying solely on vegetables, nuts and grains for your protein, you need to mix the types of plant-based food you eat. Rice and beans, for example, will do the trick, as will serving dhal with rice or spreading nut butter on wholemeal bread. You do need to make sure that you have protein in your diet every day, and that you are getting a complete range of essential amino acids, whether you eat animal products or not.

Meat

Meat is a good source of protein, but red meat in particular is also a remarkably high source of saturated fat (see page 58), which you don't want. If you want to continue to eat meat, and most people do, it is a good idea to cut back on the quantity. So go to your initial food diary (see page 32) and do a quick survey: how much meat do you actually eat in a typical week, and what sort?

Choose lean meat and poultry instead, as that will make a real difference, both to your weight-loss campaign and your general health. Another good idea is to reduce the overall quantity of meat by doing things like adding more vegetables to a stew, or substituting beans for some of the meat; they would also bring additional benefits. Chicken and turkey are great sources of comparatively low-fat protein, but note that poultry skin is also high in saturates – and in calories, of course – and non-organic chicken may be high in hormones and growth promoters. Many people are becoming increasingly concerned about animal welfare, and want to choose organic but are deterred by the cost. Instead of trying to replace everything, it might be worth trying a general reduction in the sheer quantity of meat eaten, and making sure that the meat you do use is the best possible quality. Another word of warning when it comes to considering meat as a source of protein is to beware of processed meat products, from turkey burgers to pâtés and salamis. If you eat a lot of these you would be better getting most of your protein elsewhere, as they often contain additional fat, as well as other additives such as preservatives and colourants.

Fish

Fish, on the other hand, is fabulous – not just for its protein content, though that is outstanding, but also for the beneficial fats which oily fish in particular can add to the diet (see page 57). Unlike meat, fish is low in saturated fats, and it is recommended that it should be included in the diet at least twice a week. Shellfish shares many of the same benefits and, though it can have a high cholesterol content, this does not appear to have an impact on blood-cholesterol levels. Eating more fish has been clearly associated with a reduced risk of having a heart attack, and it is also low in calories, so it has to be worth using it more. There have been some concerns about pollution and the sustainability of wild stocks, so experiment with unusual or unpopular varieties – pollack is a good substitute for cod, for instance, and fresh mackerel is not as widely used as it should be.

As with meat, don't rely on processed fish products – the protein content may still be fine, but the breadcrumbs or batter in which many are coated only provide extra calories for no nutritional benefits. Smoked fish – like smoked mackerel – is sometimes high in calories and sometimes not; smoked salmon is a good choice.

Eggs

Eggs should form part of your diet, whether you are trying to lose weight or not, because they are packed with nutrients. As a source of protein, they have all the essential amino acids in exactly the right proportions, and are actually used as the standard against which other food is assessed. There's no need to worry about their cholesterol content, either, as dietary cholesterol has little or no effect on the amount of cholesterol in the blood (that's unless you have been expressly told to avoid eggs). They are also comparatively low in calories, although they are very easy to add calories to, as they are often fried or become part of something which is high in calories, such as a quiche.

Dairy products

The problem with seeing dairy products as a source of protein is that many dairy foods are also a source of fats, and those are often saturated. Full-cream milk, for example, isn't just higher in calories; it's higher in saturated fats. But do not be tempted to cut out dairy, unless you have a medically diagnosed problem which makes it necessary, as you would be restricting your intake of a vital mineral – calcium. Cutting it out could result in reduced bone density as your body would have to draw the calcium it needed from your bones instead; but you could also be doing something totally counter-productive when it comes to losing weight – because calcium actually seems to help in weight loss. Exactly how it does this is still the subject of debate, but it is linked to an increased breakdown of fat in the body and to increased removal, rather than storage, of fat. Calcium does come from other sources, such as the bones you eat when you have sardines, or leafy green vegetables, but that from dairy food appears to be the most effective here.

Generally, when it comes to dairy products, check out the lower-fat options. But do be wary; some, particularly things like fruit yoghurts, may be high in sugar to give them some taste in compensation for the lack of fat. By the way, probiotic yoghurts may seem to be a healthy option but many are startlingly high in sugar; the same applies to the small probiotic yoghurt drinks. They are highly processed, as 'functional foods' are, and one little 100g pot can contain as much as 18g of sugar – which illustrates the importance of reading labels. Take another fruit-flavoured one: this time it has 11.3 per cent sugars. When you look at the ingredients, which are listed in order, you find that the first ones are yoghurt and skimmed milk, which is to be expected, but the next is straight sugar, 8.4 per cent. Then comes the fruit – 2.1 per cent – and that's followed by dextrose (more sugar) and flavouring. This is also a useful reminder that not all things which might appear to be 'healthy' actually are. Some Belgian research has shown that many of these quick-shot probiotic drinks didn't contain all the 'good bacteria' they were supposed to, a finding which was echoed in tests in the UK. And the effect of these bacteria, when they are there, still has to be independently researched in full, but the initial results aren't promising. There's a word of warning for all 'functional' foods, too: because they are classed as foods and not medicines, they are not subject to the same rigorous and independent checks on their claims – as yet.

When it comes to milk itself, you should be using skimmed milk or changing over to it, something which can be done gradually if you find it difficult at first. As with sugar, once you have become used to the taste of skimmed milk, you will begin to find full-cream milk (and maybe cream itself) unpleasant. And there's actually slightly *less* calcium in whole milk, too. Finally, milk which comes from grass-fed cows, which is usually organic, is naturally higher in omega-3s than that from industrially reared animals, which are often kept indoors.

Cheese can be less straightforward than milk itself. There are low-fat versions of Cheddar around but you may well find them leathery and unappealing. One solution is to use the same cheese you usually do (unexceptional often equals sustainable), but to use less and buy a stronger version – mature Cheddar rather than mild, for instance, will compensate in flavour for what you have cut in quantity. There are also some perfectly standard products which are naturally lower in fat and calories, and don't discount the traditional favourite, cottage cheese. Ricotta, another fresh cheese, and fromage frais are both naturally lower in calories than either hard cheese or crème fraîche, though they're not exactly comparable in the case of ricotta – but you could use feta which is also lower. However, not all hard cheeses are the same; Edam, for instance, is lower in calories than Cheddar. If you need help making choices, read the labels and compare calorie values per 100g.

Drinks

When you are planning a healthy diet that will help you lose weight, you need to think quite clearly about what you drink, because it can make a big difference.

We all need to drink, and it is recommended that we try to have the equivalent of six to eight glasses of water a day. This can include herb tea and some schemes allow a little ordinary tea or coffee in the count. If you are tempted by flavoured mineral waters, check the ingredients – they often have high levels of sugar.

Fizzy drinks and fruit juice

On the cold drink front, many fizzy drinks are basically sugary water with added flavourings, often artificial, and will do nothing for you other than raise blood-sugar levels and help you gain weight. 'Diet' versions of fizzy drinks often contain sugar substitutes which you'd be better off not consuming too. Most researchers come down on the side of not recommending artificial sweeteners for many reasons, mostly connected with safety and/or unpleasant side-effects. A recent study produced an interesting result – that the use of sweeteners was actually associated with weight *gain*. More work needs to be done, but the suggestion is that using such sweeteners stops people associating a sweet taste with high calorie levels, so that it is harder to subconsciously – or even consciously – regulate food intake. It does have to be said that previous studies have been inconclusive, but sugar substitutes should still be approached with caution.

Fruit juices can have an instant effect on blood sugar as there's no fibre to slow down digestion, and the same also applies to smoothies. Quicker digestion also means that you absorb fewer nutrients, so you can only count one smoothie or glass of juice against your five-a-day fruit and vegetable target.

Tea and coffee

With tea or coffee, watch the added sugar and milk. Cut back to skimmed milk – this can be done gradually, reducing from full-cream to semi-skimmed and then to fully skimmed – and be open-minded about alternatives, not just taking your coffee or tea black, though that helps. Try herb or fruit teas and experiment; there are so many varieties available now that there's bound to be something you like. Reduce the quantity of sugar, if you take it, and try to get to a point where you no longer need any; artificial sweeteners have had a bad press in the past, when it comes to the effects they can have, and some continue to do so (see above). Tea and simple coffee are not the only hot drink options, of course, and there is no way that hot chocolate piled high with cream and topped with marshmallows forms part of any sort of healthy diet on a regular basis. Be careful about the type of coffee you drink if you do take it with milk (there's a wealth of difference between an Americano with skimmed and a cappuccino with full-cream milk) and if you are tempted into buying cappuccino mixes, do read the ingredients and nutritional information panels and bear in mind that you have to add milk on top.

Alcohol

Alcohol can be a minefield. If you are drinking in a bar, you can be roughly sure of how much you are having, but do choose the smallest option when it comes to the size of glass. At parties, heaven only knows how much you're getting; the same applies to other people's homes and, unfortunately, it can also apply to your own home. Glass sizes have increased a lot over the last few years, so check your favourite wine glass and see how much it actually holds. The standard pub measure used to be 125ml; that is hardly ever the case now, and most domestic wine glasses are also larger. It's worth checking this because of the easily forgotten difference in calorie content, let alone alcohol content. The old measure – 125ml – of red wine, for instance, is 85 calories. More common now is 175ml (that often counts as a 'small' glass these days) which would be 119, and 250ml glasses are not infrequent – for which, double the calories of the old standard measure.

These are 'empty calories'; they bring you no nutritional benefits and bump up your alcohol intake without you really noticing. In addition, many wines are stronger than they were – 13.5 per cent alcohol by volume is not uncommon – and though that won't necessarily have much of an impact on your calorie intake as such, it will certainly affect your willpower.

You don't have to stop drinking when you're trying to lose weight if you like a regular glass of wine or a tot of whisky in the evening but, like everything else, keep tabs on quantity. It's worth considering that alcohol can actually slow down your body's use of fat. If alcohol is available as a source of energy – like glucose, it is digested very quickly in the stomach; think how easily you get drunk if you haven't eaten – then your body won't make use of anything else until it has used up the energy from the alcohol first.

How much should you eat?

Working out precise calorie intake for achieving weight loss is actually more complicated than you might think, given the basic fact that you'll put on weight if you take in more energy than you use, and lose it if you use more than you take in. Human bodies are not machines, and there are a lot of variables. There are plenty of sweeping generalisations around – most usually, that you should eat 1,500 calories a day if you're female and 2,000 if you're male in order to lose weight – but they are as imprecise as some of the methods of judging ideal weights. At the beginning, at least, settle for making small but gradually increasing changes to three things: what you eat, how much you eat and what you do. We've covered the first, though there's more information coming up, and that's true of the last one, too. Time to look at the middle one in more detail.

Firstly, think in terms of three meals – breakfast, lunch and supper – and a couple of snacks, keeping them all as healthy as possible. Then, portion size is key. We've all become used to larger portions than we used to have in the past – research has shown that they have increased by a third, on average – and in some places gigantic portions are now the norm (so, often, is obesity: think of parts of the US). This easily leads to over-consumption – there's a natural tendency to try and clear a plate, and it's also been noted that people who are heavier tend to give themselves bigger helpings. Serving size really can make a profound difference, potentially more than doubling the calorie cost of a meal. What is needed is a shortcut to getting the quantities and proportions roughly right, and one that will work in practice.

There are various 'healthy eating pyramids' showing the relative proportions of different foods which would make up an ideal diet, but they are better on the page than in the kitchen. No generalisation is going to be perfect, but think of a plate instead. For a traditional meal, about half the plate should be devoted to vegetables or a salad, a quarter to potatoes or rice or even pasta, and a quarter to meat or other protein. None of these should be piled so high that they would be in danger of falling off (with the exception of vegetables, if they were cooked and served in the healthiest possible way, and salads served without high-calorie dressings).

Many meals probably don't look like that nowadays, but you can use this idea and expand on it as a general guide. First, eat more vegetables and fruit than anything else, and if you are eating a meal which is based on pasta, for instance, make sure you have less pasta and a large salad. The maximum portion size for dishes like this – say pasta with pesto –

is really 100g dry weight per person, and this also applies to couscous, rice, noodles, etc., though you may find that about 80g is sufficient. If these are used as an accompaniment, you'll need much less. Try and restrict yourself to two or three slices of bread a day, as well.

Next, after fruit and vegetables, go for whole-grain, unrefined carbohydrates such as pasta, rice and wholemeal bread, but in lower quantities; don't overdo it and make sure, when you look back at your day, that you didn't concentrate on these. Then comes the largely protein element – fish, meat, dairy products – which should be eaten in moderation, concentrating on the best possible choices. The lowest quantities of all in your overall diet should be the straight oils and fats – and sugar. If you are unsure about portion sizes and high-calorie items like cheese or oil, measure if you need to until you get a feel for what a teaspoon of oil (about 45 calories) looks like in a pan, as opposed to a tablespoon (three times that).

At present official guidelines are that carbohydrate should form between 45–50 per cent of the whole; protein should be up to 15 per cent and fat a maximum of 35 per cent (though the WHO recommend that this should be 30 per cent). This figure, of course, includes the fat contained in other things, such as the 10 per cent per 100g in a steak, the 17 per cent in the same weight of cooked mackerel and the 3 per cent in plain yoghurt. Getting hung up on this would make your life difficult, not to say impractical and unsustainable, so just bear the basic order above in mind: mostly fruit and vegetables, then whole-grain carbs, then sensible protein, and finally fats and oils. Yes, you need a range of micronutrients too, but if you are eating a varied, balanced and healthy diet you'll be getting what you need without worrying too much about them in particular.

Should you wish to get more pernickety, there are all sorts of precise guidelines to portion control – never have a piece of fish bigger than a playing card, cut a piece of cheese about the size of a small matchbox and you'll be fine – but they're not really necessary. Get the proportions right, as described above, and don't go mad with high-fat, high-calorie items. Above all, go for the balance; don't let your diet swing too far towards one of the food groups because the human body needs an all-round balance of nutrients from a variety of vegetables and fruit, pulses, whole grains, fish, lean meat, the best kind of fats and some dairy produce. Something like toast for breakfast, a brown rice salad with a bread roll at lunchtime and a plate of pasta for supper should ring a few alarm bells if it happened on a regular basis. Don't eat too much of anything at the expense of other kinds of food, no matter how healthy it is.

One trick which has been used by many successful dieters when monitoring their food intake is to keep a written record, rather like the food diary at the start (page 32). You shouldn't have to weigh or count calories at this stage, not if you're keeping control of portion sizes and proportions, but jot things down and try not to forget anything. Some people have even found that photographing their meals can help. It may sound rather mad, but it could be a useful check on portion size (and it makes you think, too, before you eat).

If you find your weight-loss efforts stalling or just not happening when you eat more healthily and watch your portion sizes, you can use the 1,500 or 2,000 calories per day as a guideline to see if what you think you are eating really *is* what you are eating and is therefore going to have the effect you hope. Get a calorie guide like *Perfect Calorie Counting*, a companion book to this one, and do some weighing and measuring, because portion sizes do have a tendency to slip. In short, try and keep your approach to portion control instinctive and almost automatic, but monitored, backed up with bursts of counting if necessary. Think about the long term and you'll understand why – and who wants to be trying to find small matchboxes to measure their cheese against, anyway?

Shopping and food labelling

It all starts with buying food. When you are shopping, remember the basic rules of healthy eating, avoid the processed food and ready meals as much as you can and always check labels. Most packaged food – and no matter how 'good' you are being, there will always be some – has some nutritional information on it.

Labels can be amazingly informative, but they can also be amazingly misleading – if you let them. At the very least there should be an ingredients list, and the thing to know about these is that the ingredients are listed in order of how much the product contains. So if 'sugar' is at the top, there's more sugar in it than anything else. You'll be able to recognise many of the ingredients, but if you can't – long chemical names or E-numbers will also be listed – it's probably best to treat this as a sign that you should look for an alternative. Many products also have nutritional information panels, listing things like protein content as a percentage per 100g (and often also per portion; ignore this, as manufacturers' ideas of what constitutes a portion are very variable). These can give you a good idea of how healthy something really is – check out some 'healthy' or 'diet' ready meals; they can be quite entertaining.

Some labelling in the UK gives a proportion of the 'guideline daily amount' (GDA) for a particular nutritional element – such as salt, protein or sugar – that a product contains, and these figures are usually found on the front of the package, in a relatively prominent position; they may be in different colours. GDAs are a food industry measure which attempt to make the rest of the nutritional labelling easier to understand, but it's better to go straight to the nutrition labels instead. They are more objective than the GDAs, which you can afford to ignore as they are not always clear and can even be misleading – the most common problem is that the portion sizes used are not always relevant. To take one example, a can of fizzy drink may cite GDAs for 100ml of product, but the can contains 330ml. Anyone drinking the cola or lemon or whatever would be likely to drink the whole can rather than measure out 100ml (not a lot), so they would actually be drinking more than three times the quantities on the GDA panel. GDA figures are usually also for adults, even on children's food lines. So stick with those ingredients lists and nutritional information panels.

It's worth looking at what labelling around fat really means, too. In the EU, if something is labelled as being 'fat-free' it has to have less than 0.5g fat per 100g, and a 'low-fat' product has less than 3g fat per 100g. If something is called 'reduced fat', then it must contain at least 25 per cent less fat than a standard equivalent (which could, of course, mean it is still high in fat). Do bear in mind that products that are low in fat are often high in sugars, to compensate for the reduced taste, so check out the full nutritional information panels anyway.

As a final note here, don't buy anything you really hate just because you think it might be good for your overall diet. If you loathe Brussels sprouts, don't buy them just because they're loaded with goodies; leave the little horrors in the shop. If you think crispbread is no better than cardboard, then don't eat it; it's not obligatory just because it's long been associated with dieting. Don't punish yourself – think sustainable instead, and take a balanced approach.

Cooking

It is easy to make small adaptations that will have a very big effect when you are preparing food, so here's how to begin. As you progress, you will inevitably find that you will start making your own adaptations too.

As a shortcut when cooking, think of grilling, baking, poaching, steaming, boiling or microwaving most of the time, before you think about cooking anything in a way which would require a lot of additional calories – frying, basically. Frying adds fat to whatever you're cooking, and deep-frying adds a lot, so the most obvious thing to do is to ditch the deep-fryer, if you have one.

Using non-stick pans is an easy way of making a positive change, as you don't need very much oil or fat when using them and can safely reduce the quantities in recipes without it affecting the taste too much. Occasional frying is fine if you use that non-stick pan, choose the right kind of oil, measure the amount and use as little as possible, and blot whatever you have fried on kitchen paper to take off any excess. Some things – bacon is the best example – will cook very successfully without any additional fat at all, as they will shed a lot of their own fat, which can then be drained away. Blot dry-fried bacon on kitchen paper, and you could make a great calorie saving; grilled bacon is also good, but should also be blotted.

Stir-fries are fabulous. Not only do they require comparatively little oil, they are generally packed with nutritious ingredients – and the shorter the cooking time, the more nutrients the food retains. The other way to maximise nutrients is not to throw some of them away; they can be retained in the liquid of a soup, for instance, rather than leached into the water and emptied down the sink when you drain cooked vegetables. Casseroles are a good way to retain nutrients as well. Steaming vegetables preserves more nutrients than boiling and steamed food tends not to need any fatty additives; nor does food cooked 'en papillote' (sealed in a parcel of foil or baking paper).

If you have never measured cooking ingredients, such as oil or butter when frying, you need to start. Measure high-fat items, of which something like cheese is a classic example. Small errors and assumptions can make a big difference, and while you won't generally need to count every single calorie, you should be cutting back on those high-calorie ingredients. With cheese, for instance, stick at about 25g for a single helping. Get some good scales; a slimmer's set – which weighs smaller quantities – is useful for any cook (if you try and measure that 25g accurately on ordinary scales, you'll find out why). Another useful thing to have is a set of standard spoon measures, as ordinary spoons can vary so much. A spoon measure set should contain a standard tablespoon (15ml), teaspoon (5ml), plus half and quarter teaspoons. These are especially useful for measuring oil, as just sloshing it out of the bottle can add a lot of unnecessary calories.

Adapting ordinary recipes

There's no need to buy specialist cookery books if you are trying to lose weight. They can often be depressingly boring, and you don't want to be thinking in terms of something you might only need to do for a short while; it would be counter-productive when you're going for long-term change.

Recipes can easily be modified in most cases by reducing the quantities of fat and sugar (and salt can usually be reduced too; you might as well go for all-round health benefits). Adding fibre is a good idea as well, and more straightforward than it sounds – using more whole grains and vegetables; leaving the skins on potatoes used in dishes; adding pulses to soups, salads and casseroles; not peeling fruit. Use skimmed milk, low-fat plain yoghurt and maybe low-fat crème fraîche, which is stable over a gentle heat and can be used in cooking instead of cream. Cook with olive or rapeseed oil, and measure it – don't forget that the same measuring rule should apply to all high-calorie ingredients, as using more than you need can make a massive difference. In Chapter 8 you'll find more practical information on using specific types of food, together with examples of straightforward recipes showing how they have been adapted.

Appreciate your food and savour every mouthful; if this means eating more slowly, then so much the better. Research has shown that overweight and obese people do tend to eat more quickly. There is a real link between the rate of eating and the amount of satisfaction you get, and the more satisfied you are, the less likely you are to eat huge quantities without thinking about it. So slow down – and enjoy your food.

5 Keeping it personal

One of the most obvious things about losing weight, though you wouldn't necessarily know it from the way some diet plans are supposed to be universally applicable, is that everyone's requirements are different. It's time to consider some of these variations on the theme of weight loss and see how they can work with a balanced and sustainable approach.

Vegetarianism

If you are a vegetarian who wants to lose weight, the same rough principles apply to you as they do to everyone else – eat less, watch *what* you eat and move about more – but there are some special considerations. While a vegetarian diet can be extremely healthy, it can also be deficient in some vitamins, notably B_{12}, which is derived from animal products. It may be necessary to take a supplement, and there are vegetarian and vegan ones around. Iron can also be low, but most vegetarians are well aware of this and take measures to avoid it, such as eating more pulses and nuts. A vitamin C supplement may be useful here, as it can aid the absorption of iron from plant sources. Lacto-vegetarians (who do not eat dairy products) will probably need to take a calcium supplement; soya milk is often an alternative, but get one with added calcium.

It's often thought that vegetarians don't share the same weight problems as meat-eaters but this is not always the case, so don't decide to adopt a vegetarian diet just because you think it will help you lose weight. Vegetarians are often likely to be healthier in other ways, though, such as having lower cholesterol levels which may be partly due to generally eating less saturated fat than non-vegetarians. But there can still be too much saturated fat in a vegetarian diet if the person in question eats a lot of dairy products, and many vegetarians do have a tendency to overeat cheese (and specifically vegetarian cheese is still high in calories). Monitoring your intake of such foods is a good way to begin, and so is watching the quantity of potatoes or bread, which can also creep up. It is important to apply the same rule about avoiding refined carbohydrates, but even healthier wholemeal bread can have a bad effect if you eat too much. So can nuts, another potential danger area.

Having said that, there are some huge advantages to a good vegetarian diet and thinking like a vegetarian can be good for any dieter. Getting more than the recommended five-a-day portions of fruit and vegetables is not likely to be a problem, for instance, and most vegetarians are used to incorporating pulses in their everyday diet on a regular basis. Many also use soya, either as a meat substitute or instead of some dairy products, and that can have a variety of benefits – so many, in fact, that a 25g daily target for soya protein has been suggested for everyone. A lot of vegetarians are also more adventurous about experimenting with unfamiliar ingredients; quinoa, for example, was present in health-food shops long before it migrated into the supermarket mainstream. Cooking for yourself is quite normal when you're vegetarian, as the number of processed foods which are truly acceptable is low. Vegetarians are also more used to reading labels when shopping, as even products which look superficially fine can contain unacceptable animal derivatives.

Pregnancy – and afterwards

Pregnancy really is the last time to be thinking about trying to keep your weight down and dieting as such, though you should try not to put on too much additional weight. Ideas of how much is too much have changed over time, and how much is right for you depends on your BMI before conception, so talk to your GP or nurse.

Pregnancy is, however, a vital time to make sure you are eating healthily because good nutrition is absolutely essential, not just for you but also for the health of your baby. Follow the general guidelines about cutting out processed and junk food as much as you can, watch the amount of saturated fat in your diet and try to eliminate trans fats completely, eat more than the five-a-day guideline for fruit and vegetables and keep tabs on sugar and salt. Make sure your overall diet contains plenty of protein (you'll also need to consider this if you are breastfeeding). If you are eating a really healthy diet you should be getting the full range of vitamins and minerals that you need, but pay particular attention to calcium, iron, vitamin B_2, folic acid and vitamin C, which aids iron absorption. Try to eat lots of fresh fruit on a regular basis – for the vitamin C, particularly – and plenty of spinach, broccoli, beans and pulses, as well as a decent amount of protein, and you should be getting what you need. Keep up with the whole grains to ensure that your diet contains plenty of fibre, as that will help to offset the constipation which many women experience during the late stages of pregnancy.

You also need to ensure that your diet is as varied as possible, and that you aren't sliding into any habitual eating patterns which could undermine it. Most pregnant women suffer from cravings at some point, and they can be unusual or quite ordinary (pickled cucumber and olives with jam versus apples). The ones to watch out for are those which could damage your healthy eating plan because they are high in salt, fat or sugar. There's a popular feeling that your body is craving these because you have somehow become deficient in them, but there isn't any clear scientific evidence to support this idea, although hormones do play some sort of role. If you can work out what is going on when you begin to feel the urge to eat a whole pack of onion bagels, then you are half way to controlling it; think about your craving before you give in and keep a note. You may well find that boredom is a trigger, so distract yourself as much as possible. Check out the section on cravings too (see page 83).

When it comes to exercise, moderate it if you were previously into gym sessions or running, and stick to walking and swimming in the later stages. Some vigorous exercise can have a negative effect on your baby's bone density, so do take advice – and you must definitely do that if you have a history of miscarriage or problems in early pregnancy. But whatever you do, don't use your pregnancy as a reason to eat what you want and do nothing!

Losing weight after the birth of a child can seem daunting, a prospect not helped by coverage of scarily thin celebrity mothers and a lot of stress on 'getting back in shape' in the media. But everyone is different; some of those scary people will have had elective Caesareans, may have been Photoshopped anyway and will almost certainly have had personal trainers breathing down their necks. They are also quite likely to have been eating ridiculously little, and there's no need for the rest of us to follow their example at all. Do not try and do everything at once or assume you are a failure; the chances are that you're a lot healthier than the post-baby stick insects, anyway. Just remember there are three things you should do: keep to a healthy diet, do some moderate exercise and breastfeed. Finally, a few years ago some publicity was given to the discovery of a gene which seemed to be linked to whether or not women lost weight easily after pregnancy. It doesn't mean you are condemned to never losing the weight you gained if you do carry this gene, as the negative effects of possessing it can be overcome by doing two hours of regular exercise a week.

Feeding a family

If you are following a freaky diet, it is almost impossible for you to enjoy a normal life of any kind. On the other hand, if you are eating healthily but simply eating less so that you lose some weight, it is perfectly possible. It is also important not to feel isolated when you are trying to shed some excess weight – imagine how you would feel if you sat at the table eating lettuce while everyone else enjoyed a large meal, and you'll soon appreciate the difference in sustainability.

The general healthy eating rules apply to family food, but you may need to make some adaptations; after all, not everyone may need to lose weight and you should consider children's requirements. It's all in portion sizes and accompaniments. Keep your own portion sizes sensible and don't have more than a spoonful of any high-calorie extras. If there is something you find difficult to resist you may need to make more radical changes, but start gently and see how you manage. Again it's a question of balance and sustainability: make your weight-loss effort exceptional and it will fail. You need to make it as easy as possible for you to succeed, so adapt accordingly. There are foods, for example, which you may want to avoid even though other members of the family may enjoy them, such as gravy or cream. When you are cooking, ensure that these can be served separately or added afterwards rather than being part of the dish itself, and there should be no problem.

Children

On a general level, childhood obesity is definitely increasing. Barely a day goes by without some alarming statistic in the press, or a story about this or that official recommendation which is supposed to help. It isn't an imaginary state of affairs and it is a serious one, because overweight and obese children are likely to become overweight and obese adults who will require more medical treatment and live less long than their leaner contemporaries – or, in fact, than their parents. As a result, if you think your child is in danger of becoming part of these statistics, it is all too easy to panic and impose a strict diet which will usually fail, generally because you can't control everything your kids eat. But children and young people are not adults, and their requirements are different, so the first thing to do is stop, think and assess the situation calmly and realistically.

There are many considerations when it comes to trying to do something about a child's weight, and the most fundamental is whether or not that child really has a problem. It may seem obvious to you, but there are several things to think about. Children do not grow at a steady pace and, particularly in adolescence, an apparent weight problem can be resolved by the next growth spurt. You cannot use adult BMI tables with children – well, with anyone under the age of 18 – as they are still growing, and that distorts the picture. Another thing to think about is your own perception, which might lead you to believe there is a problem when there isn't. So if you find yourself worrying about a particular child, talk to your GP for an impartial view. The doctor will be able to apply the extremely variable paediatric BMI charts (there are some available online and in reference books, but there are a lot of elements to be considered, and it would not be wise to make a judgement based entirely on these), and may well get you to monitor the situation over a few months. Another thing to beware of is the other side of the coin: believing that there is no difficulty when there is. Do try and be objective, and try not to be offended if a disinterested party such as a teacher mentions a problem to you which you do not think is serious. Talk to someone else – your doctor is a good place to start. A formal diet, however, is not.

Obsessing about a child's weight has been shown to lead to either rebellion, depression or an equal obsession on the part of the child – and that raises the spectre of eating disorders. Even weighing children can be misleading because of their growth spurts; play it by ear and don't push too much. Simple healthy eating and more activity can make a real difference, but healthy eating for an adult and healthy eating for a child are not quite the same. Children, particularly young children, should not have too much fibre, for example, as it can prevent them from absorbing other nutrients. Nor should small children be having skimmed or semi-skimmed milk; growing kids need more energy. It is particularly important that they receive the full range of nutrients, so never, ever, contemplate any of the restrictive diets if you are worried about a child's weight. What you can do, without any worries at all about depriving them of necessary nutrients, is get rid of the junk. Fast food, crisps, sweets and sugary rubbish, and – this is really important – sugary drinks.

The main source of excess sugars in the diet of most children is soft drinks, canned and otherwise (they are also a significant source for many adults). Of course there are others, such as all that confectionery and cheap chocolate, biscuits, preserves and even breakfast cereals and cereal bars. Cereals designed specifically for children are often amazingly high in sugar; it's another reason to check those labels; just because they may look superficially healthy, it doesn't mean they are. But back to soft drinks, fizzy and otherwise. It has been shown that teenagers who have a can of sugary drink a day are likely to be a whopping 6.4 kilos larger than those kids who don't – and that's after only one year. You can swap standard versions for 'diet' ones, but your overall aim should be to get rid of them altogether, or to do so as much as you can. Keep the more unhealthy food and drink out of the house, as that automatically makes it less easy to get, especially if your children come home before you do – prime snacking time. Do remember that you really cannot control every single thing your child eats or drinks, but if you can remove the majority of the undesirables you will be doing a great job, and that applies to canned drinks as much as it does to sweets and crisps.

There's another source of excess sugar to think about. If you're feeding a baby, watch out for it in baby food. This is especially important because some researchers believe that early exposure to refined sugars can get children 'hooked on sweetness' right at the point when they would normally be being weaned away from it. It's worth making your own purées, and there are plenty of books and websites out there with suggestions to help.

With children, activity is one area where even a little can make a difference, and one of the most important things you can do is find something to replace a lot of the time your child spends in front of a screen. It's common sense, really, but several studies – recent ones have come from the US and New Zealand – have shown that larger children watch more television or spend longer at a computer. It's partly the inactivity, but watching more TV also means watching many more advertisements for food and drink, as well as any which are 'embedded' in the programmes (and they are not usually ads for healthy food), so do cut screen time. There's another factor, too – reducing the TV time of the children in the US study made an immediate impact simply in terms of them eating fewer calories. They just weren't snacking as much any more, and the snacks they did eat were much healthier; lower in sugar, fat and salt. That's particularly impressive because it was an unconscious and unplanned change, a simple side-effect of just watching less television.

As a final note, this has to be a family effort. Nobody could really be expected to tackle their food and activity issues if the rest of the family were carrying on as before, eating whole cakes and watching DVDs all evening without making any movement. Reinstate family mealtimes as far as is possible, and never eat 'in passing' or in front of the TV, but around a table where you can talk to each other; this will slow down eating and, as a result, help everyone feel more satisfied. Children, especially young ones but older ones as well, will tend to imitate the adults around them without necessarily realising that they are doing so. Make sure you are worth imitating, without nagging, and you'll be helping yet again. Kids are also often keen to help with cooking, so why not encourage them to do so, at least some of the time? If they can learn to cook from you, they'll have a skill which will help them all their lives, and if you're not a confident cook, you can learn together.

6 Keeping control

No weight-loss scheme ever goes entirely according to plan. You cannot anticipate everything, but you can deal with situations when they arise, and you can accommodate special circumstances. Everyone who tries to lose weight has problems at some point, whether that's simply a desire to eat a whole packet of biscuits in a sitting or give up completely. And when you do get to the weight you want to be, maintaining it can also seem difficult. An essential point, though, is to not let anything like this stress you out, but to stay calm. There's always a way through.

Moments of weakness

All dieters experience difficulties, or have periods when they fail to lose weight or even put some back on. And most dieters will feel hungry at some point, though with a truly healthy diet this shouldn't be too much of a problem. Some glitches are comparatively minor, like weight-loss stalling or the desire to eat several packets of peanuts at one go, while others – such as wanting to give up or feeling yourself slide into a pattern of bingeing – can have a greater impact. The most useful thing is to recognise what is going on, because problems can be overcome.

Stalling and gaining

Weight loss never, ever follows a smooth downwards curve, no matter how virtuous you are, but it can still seem depressing when your weight loss stalls and you hit a plateau or when you even gain a little. It *will* happen, so anticipate it and don't worry too much. Everyone experiences this, and stalls and gains are two of the reasons why some people prefer not to weigh themselves – if they don't know that they've failed to lose another half kilo this week, or even put one back on, they can't fret about it. The most important thing to do is not to worry and to carry on regardless as long as the overall trend is in the right direction. It's important to realise that there are perfectly normal fluctuations in weight. If you've stalled, do not be tempted into trying a starvation diet to get things moving again, because it won't work – yes, you might lose a bit at the time, but it will come back.

One of the most helpful things you can do in either of these circumstances is go back to writing things down. It's not that much of a chore and can make a difference all by itself. If it doesn't, then at least you've got a written record to check through and see where you might be going astray. Your occasional treats might have become rather less occasional; your consumption of bread might have sneaked upwards; you might have been having more to drink than you thought. Make sure you're not slipping back into your old habits, too – have biscuits reappeared in the cupboard? Have they been finished over the course of a week? And even healthy food can provide too many calories if there's too much of it, of course. You may well be eating more than you think you are, so do some weighing and measuring for a more objective check. And go back to portion sizes – they have a tendency to creep upwards – and think about yours. Have they become larger, and not so healthily balanced? Maybe you're still piling your plate too high, or maybe it's the opposite: you're just not eating enough and your body is – basically – hanging on to what it's got. If you are also suffering from headaches, a general unexplained tiredness and weakness that could be the case, but those are all fairly extreme symptoms of undereating. Try and be objective, and checking your consumption will help you to be just that. If you are eating at around the right level, carry on.

Another strategy is to accept a stall and use it. Take a break from trying to lose more weight and just make sure you don't add any; give your body time to adapt before you get cracking again.

Hunger

If you find yourself getting hungry, then checking what, and when, you are eating will help. If you are eating three balanced meals and having two healthy snacks, you should not be feeling that hungry. Perhaps you have slipped into a routine where you are missing out on a proper breakfast; time to get back to that. Your mid-afternoon snack might have become a few sweet biscuits, which will raise your blood-sugar levels quickly only for you to experience the effects of an equally sudden drop.

You could also be eating too little. Make sure you are not doing this by checking your calorie intake – weigh, measure and write down for a week, and make sure you are not eating fewer than 1,500 calories or thereabouts if you are female, 2,000 if you are male. You should never need to go more than 250 calories below these figures, and don't contemplate even that on a regular basis; your body needs a full range of nutrients and that is difficult to achieve if you are not eating enough.

Cravings

There are times when it cannot be denied: you really, really want to eat something, you know it's not what you should be eating and that it's going to be bad for your diet. Well, you could try and ignore it, but that will probably not work. A good way of dealing with a savoury craving is to have a small snack with a powerful savoury punch, something like Marmite on an oatcake or a piece of crispbread. Check out anchovy pastes, too – these are so strong that you couldn't possibly overindulge. If you are craving cake, have a slice of fruit loaf. Many of these are fat free, containing lots of dried fruit, so are better than most alternatives, even if they aren't low in calories. That advantage would be negated, however, if you covered your fruit loaf in butter. And do stop at one slice or a single oatcake; not doing so could set off a binge.

Cravings are more likely to occur when your blood-sugar levels are low, so keep them as steady as you can by eating regularly: three meals and two healthy snacks during the course of a day.

A sweet tooth

Having a really sweet tooth can be a problem, but it is one that can be solved. In the long term, you need to think about reducing your need for sugary foods, and you may well find that one of the best ways of doing this is going cold turkey: cut it out. There will still be sweetness in your normal diet, but not the extra sugar that you have been adding on top. It is difficult, but losing or reducing a sweet tooth can be done. One of the reasons why it can be so hard to reduce the taste for sugar in practice is that it has become so universal in prepared foods that it's now very difficult to avoid. Sugar is included in an enormous variety of products, from breakfast cereals to savoury biscuits, and it is used to bulk things up as well as provide extra taste which would otherwise be lacking due to poor or depleted ingredients. So, yet again, cut back the amount of processed and prepared food that you buy and, once you have done that, look at the sugar you voluntarily add to your food and drink and reduce that too. And remember it's a sweet tooth you're dealing with – so replacing sugar with artificial sweeteners is not going to solve the problem (see page 63 for more information on why sugar substitutes aren't a good idea).

Bingeing and disordered eating

Everyone who tries to lose weight will probably binge at some time, but it's a lot more likely if you're following a hard-line restrictive 'diet' than if you are just eating healthily – yet another reason for avoiding such diets completely. Boredom and binges are very often linked. In addition, some women find that they're more susceptible to binges at certain times of the month. Binges are also connected to feelings of frustration and anger – but here you need to realise that eating a 250g bar of chocolate in one go isn't going to change anything; it will just make you feel worse. It's time to break the pattern, to examine the reasons for your feelings and to do something about them.

There are several strategies you can employ if a binge is looming. The most effective is distraction when you can tell one is about to happen – just do something, anything, to take your attention away from food. Exercise is great for this, so go for a walk. If exercise is not practical, there will be some other way you can take your mind off a possible binge. If you're at work, giving in will most likely be either impractical or embarrassing, so use that to put you off – do you really want your boss to see you scarfing a whole pack of biscuits? Can you really dash out of the office and buy a giant bag of crisps? In reality the answer is likely to be no, so go for another form of distraction. Do something that you either know will absorb your attention completely or take you into direct contact with other people.

If you are in the house late at night and the fridge is calling you, it may be less easy to avoid the call – unless you have ensured that your fridge only contains healthy food and that you have frozen anything potentially naughty, like leftover fruit crumble. Binges usually need immediate satisfaction, so if something has to be defrosted, it's no good. You could distract yourself with a hot drink and a really good DVD, or do something with your hands like playing cards, surfing the Internet or joining the craft revival and knitting. Try a lovely hot bath with lots of bubbles, or go to bed with a good book. Whatever you do, remember that tomorrow is another day.

If you find that binges are happening regularly, then take a look at your diet as a whole. There is a chance that you may be eating too little, so keep a meticulous food diary – and this time weigh things. Your sliver of cheese may be 50g, not the 10g you assumed it was. Or is it more of a binge sparked by a craving? Have you eliminated something you actually love eating? Take a look at it, and see if you can incorporate whatever it is without going overboard. Both binges and cravings can be the result of leaving too long a gap between meals, so make sure that's not the problem. Or maybe you've just cut out too much at once and are trying to change the world. Which leads to the real warning: if you've had a bingey day, do not, under any circumstances whatsoever, try and cut down on what you eat the following day to compensate. That will make the situation worse. Just carry on as normal.

Binges can, of course, slide into eating disorders and if you feel this is happening to you, seek professional help. You don't have to see your

GP if you don't want to, but you should talk to somebody. In the UK, the Eating Disorders Association can be very helpful (see page 156).

Giving up

One common reaction to something like a binge is the desire to give up – the 'Well, I've blown it so what's the point?' argument. This is very common and one single thing can often lead to the abandonment of a whole weight-loss effort. Guard against this possibility happening to you. Just get back on your diet rather than walking away from every-thing you have achieved. Losing any weight at all is a great achievement, so value it and don't trash it because you're feeling fed up; hang on in there. You can learn from the experience, too, so that you won't be tempted into this reaction if it happens again.

If you feel like giving up in other circumstances, then consider the possibility seriously and try to work out why. Changing a lifestyle is not something that can be done in a flash, whatever the impression that cer-tain television programmes may give. You may have been trying to do too much, too fast; slow down. You may have been trying to speed the process along by eating abnormally; stop. You may have been eating a lot of the same thing and become bored; vary what you're eating more. And, as above, think about the weight you have already lost: do you really want that to come back on? Try to recall why you wanted to lose weight in the first place, and also think about how you have been mon-itoring your weight loss. If you made a note of your starting weight, find it and realise how far you have come; if you had a pair of previously very snug jeans, try them on. Everyone experiences phases when they can't be bothered, but that's all it is – a phase.

Giving up can be encouraged by friends and family in ways which might be well-meant but which are none the less unnerving. When someone begins to change physically it can be unsettling for others – the fundamental nature of your relationships can appear to change. Maybe you were always the safe one to be with when the gang was out on the town, because you were no threat; maybe your partner suddenly realises that other people might be finding you attractive; maybe there's some simple jealousy from those of your friends who are larger than you, or maybe your mother is worried that 'all this losing weight is making you miserable'. You can't deal with other people's problems, well-intentioned or not; you can only deal with your own. So think clearly about your reasons for wanting to walk away and make sure they're not based on pressure from other people.

Maybe what you need is a break or some encouragement. Don't slip back into old habits, but reward yourself with something new – how about a luxury weekend away or a sauna session or a trip somewhere you've always wanted to go? Maybe you could just forget the 'diet' (of course, thinking of it in these terms could be part of the problem) and enjoy a meal out with friends and family. Have a pause.

Disrupted routines

One of the most important things to bear in mind is that the key to success and sustainability is to make things as easy as possible, so do not put your willpower to impossible tests. Apply this thinking when you are looking at the prospect of something like a holiday or celebration disrupting your diet. When you are losing weight you can still enjoy the sort of events that you would have enjoyed if you had not been dieting, so you can – and must – continue to do things like eating out and celebrating with friends and family. The more trying to lose weight becomes an unusual and penitential undertaking, the less weight you are likely to lose and keep off in the long term.

Eating out

If your diet really is sustainable, then you can cope with eating out. You shouldn't create abnormal conditions when you're trying to lose weight, and for many of us 'abnormal conditions' would mean never eating out. Do not, however, be tempted into starving yourself in anticipation, or cutting down drastically the following day. There are some basic guidelines, in addition to those about healthy eating and portion control, and you will find some useful tips in the last chapter too. How strictly you apply the guidelines will depend on how frequently you eat out. If you have a curry every Friday, then you'll need to be quite firm; confine yourself to a tandoori or tikka (not a tikka masala, note) with a salad, rather than a dish with a lot of high-calorie sauce, mountains of rice and a stuffed naan. If you visit your local curry house infrequently, you could afford that tikka masala or lamb dupiaza but would still be best advised to cut back on the rice and avoid anything deep-fried like samosas.

So, in brief, and in addition to general healthy eating:
- Ask questions about ingredients if you need to.
- Don't fill up on bread while you are reading the menu.
- Eat slowly, really appreciating what you are eating.
- Eat more vegetables than anything else, but be careful about sauces and dressings for salads. You can ask for them to be served separately.
- Avoid fried food as far as possible, and particularly anything which has been deep-fried (that includes chips, of course); cream, as far as possible; thick sauces; and pastry.
- Think twice before you order dessert.
- Cheese is not necessarily a better choice than dessert when it comes to calories. Either have coffee instead or ask for fresh fruit. But be wary of fruit salads, as they may be made with sugar syrup, and if you do choose one, don't add cream.
- Only drink alcohol while you are actually eating.

Being entertained

When you are eating at someone else's house it is not quite so easy to follow the eating-out guidelines, though you can still apply several of them, like avoiding bread and only drinking when you are eating. What you do not have is control of the menu, but you are – generally – able to control your portion sizes and the relative proportions of what you eat so, again, make it more vegetables than anything else. But events like this are unlikely to be the norm, so allow yourself some latitude; think balanced and sustainable and don't get hung up on trying to achieve the impossible.

When it comes to parties, you are on much more shifting ground. What food there is will probably be fairly unhealthy, and there is also likely to be a plentiful supply of alcohol – not a good combination. You have two choices, essentially: to let yourself go completely or to try and restrain yourself as much as you can. Again the saving grace is that parties are probably not going to be that regular an event. You'll find more party survival tips in the final chapter (see page 149) but two useful ones to start with are never to turn up at a party feeling hungry (have something to eat beforehand) and to begin by drinking water (you can tell people it's vodka if you wish). If you avoid going to parties you are turning your weight-loss campaign into something abnormal again. Go, enjoy yourself, and get back on the wagon the next day.

Celebrations, holidays and religious festivals

Christmas and other religious festivals are often difficult for anyone trying to lose weight and so are other celebrations, such as weddings, where food features and the menu is out of your control. The best thing to do is to give yourself some time off from your weight-loss routine; the flexibility of eating healthily and just eating less means that it should be perfectly possible for you to enjoy special events without them causing too much pain or having too great an impact on your diet. But it is just time off and not a reason to stop completely. Nor is it a licence to throw caution to the winds, eat an entire box of chocolates and follow it with half a ton of Brazil nuts, but do not try and be a martyr when everyone else is enjoying themselves either. That would be just as counter-productive, and more likely to lead to excessive chocolate consumption.

Allow up to week for a major celebration like Christmas and the odd day off for other events like Easter or a family wedding, plus a couple of days for your birthday. Avoid giving yourself time off too often because you need to leave some leeway for holidays.

When you are away on holiday, whether that's two weeks in the sun or a weekend city break, do not fret too much about trying to lose weight. Yes, make sure you eat healthily as much as you can, and try and ensure that you don't drink too much, but do not obsess about it. If you've been eating healthily for some time, you are likely to find that making good choices in restaurants is automatic and that you don't want a huge plateful of chips any more. You might not, of course, in which case you could go for a few chips rather than a lot. Keep treats as treats rather than holiday normality, though (what goes on tour doesn't, unfortunately, really stay on tour and you may find changing back quite difficult). Whatever you do, don't make yourself – or your companions – miserable. Holidays should be fun and your diet should be sustainable, and the two can go together very well.

Getting there – and staying there

As you diet you will want to know how you are doing and keep tabs on your progress. It can be quite difficult to motivate yourself without some form of assessment, and while encouraging remarks are helpful – there's almost nothing to beat a spontaneous, 'Wow, you're looking really good' – it would be rash to rely on them. Keeping to your target weight will also require a bit of monitoring, as well as some gentle adjustment. The trick is to find something that really works for you, both when you are losing the weight, and when you are trying to maintain your new weight.

Monitoring weight loss

There are several ways to monitor the progress of your weight-loss effort, and one of the most obvious is weighing yourself. However, some people find that this does not help at all and can even be a disincentive – they can have a strong reaction to the small losses, stalls and occasional gains which are normal parts of a long-term strategy. It is possible that you think you are fine with weighing yourself until you encounter one of these situations, and then you find yourself heading for the biscuit barrel in consolation. If that sounds like you, scrap the scales. But if that isn't you at all and *you* can cope, make sure you always put the scales in the same place and wear the same clothes (preferably nothing) when you weigh yourself, and always do so at the same time of day. Remember, what you are looking for is an overall trend downwards and that weight fluctuates for all sorts of reasons. You can go by the fit of your clothes instead, but however you decide to monitor your weight loss, don't obsess about it. Expect fluctuations and then you won't be surprised when they happen. Be prepared to lose weight in stages.

Maintaining a new weight

Reaching target is often the point at which diets go astray, but these are mostly restrictive and low-calorie diets. The most important thing to do when you have reached your target is not to throw everything up in the air and abandon all your good intentions, though it can be very tempting. It is much more tempting, however, if you have been following a restrictive and temporary diet, rather than making permanent changes to your lifestyle. You are much less likely to be reckless if you have been dieting sustainably – and this is the reason why you have been trying to do just that.

The chances are that you would be most unhappy were you to be suddenly presented with the food you ate quite normally before the whole process began. On the off-chance that you are tempted to turn your back on your healthy approach, just remember that the old ways of eating are what caused the problem in the first place. What you do need to do is to stop losing more weight, however, so you should increase your calorie intake a little. Add an extra slice of wholemeal bread to your lunch, have another healthy snack during the day – build slowly and surely but keep your weight stable and your diet healthy. If you do feel tempted to go back to having a bar of chocolate on the way home, resist; it will be comparatively easy to do that, now, as well. Another element to bear in mind is that this is the point at which increased activity levels and exercise can be a real advantage, helping you maintain your new weight.

If you find things slipping – and it is probably a good idea to weigh yourself now, just to help you monitor what's happening – then cut back to your previous levels of food intake. You will soon find a stable position. Stick with it and you will soon be much, much healthier as well as lighter in weight.

7 Keeping it real – and sustainable

It can be easy to get bogged down by the theory of what you should be eating and what you should be avoiding when you are trying to lose weight and eat healthily, and putting that information into practice in the real world can sometimes seem problematic. But it doesn't have to be.

Here you will find some more basic, practical information. It's gathered into broad categories, according to basic meal types, but they are not mutually exclusive – you'll find information about bread, for instance, under 'Breakfast and brunch', though you may well eat bread at other times of the day; and there's an adapted version of mushrooms on toast there which might be good for lunch or supper, as well as being delicious for a morning meal. Within each section there is more information about good and bad choices of food and potential pitfalls. When it comes to drinks, check out pages 63–5.

This is also where to come for some initial recipes. You might assume that you are condemned to lettuce leaves and dry bread when you're trying to lose weight, but that is far from the case – remember, there's no need to be penitential. All the recipes are for perfectly normal dishes, but I'll explain how each one varies from a more conventional version, so as to demonstrate the process involved in adapting an ordinary recipe to a weight-loss programme. You'll see that this is perfectly possible; there's no need to rush out and buy slimming cookery books. All these recipes are easy and healthier – higher in nutrients and fibre, with no artificial additives – than the equivalent processed version or 'ready meal', where one exists (see pages 115–17 for more on ready meals). Seasoning has not been specified, so use salt and pepper according to your taste, where appropriate.

Finally, a word about the fat you use in cooking. Measure, measure, measure – and remember that not all oils and fats are the same when it comes to nutritional benefits, though they may have almost-identical calorie values. Generally, try not to use too much butter or ghee, but go for an oil instead wherever possible. Olive and rapeseed oils are the ones to choose most of the time, and using a spoon measure is the best way to ensure you don't use too much; they may be good for you, but a small error could still make a big difference to calorie levels. You'll find more information on pages 57–9. Serving sizes are given in the recipes.

Breakfast and brunch

Breakfast is vital. Many studies have shown a real difference in weight loss between those dieters who do have breakfast, and those who do not. Blood-sugar levels will drop during the night, and if you miss breakfast you'll most likely be hit by an urgent need to eat something, *anything*, a little later – and that's likely to be something high in calories too. A good, low-GI breakfast is the best way of keeping you going until lunch, and it doesn't have to be cereal, either: think kippers, yoghurt with fresh fruit, a boiled egg or baked beans on wholemeal toast …

Breakfast cereals

Many brands of cereal are anything but healthy, despite the fact that a lot stress their healthiness on the packaging. Always check the ingredients before buying and watch out for salt and sugar levels – they are often high. Most brands also have a high GI, so they will have a swift impact on your blood sugar and leave you feeling hungry again by mid-morning. There are some which are better than others, but in many ways you can help your diet by making your own, which is not as hippy-dippy as it sounds.

And then there's porridge. Porridge is a fantastic breakfast food, and not just for dieters; it's good for your all-round health because of the soluble fibre it contains. Oats are almost always the best choice when it comes to breakfast cereals, but buy whole oats rather than a pre-cooked 'quick' brand. The quick-cook brands are processed, partly broken down, and consequently have a higher GI than standard varieties. That means they won't be as satisfying as standard porridge, and you'll feel hungry more quickly. Ordinary porridge oats don't have to be cooked for ages, anyway, so those are definitely the ones to choose.

Orange muesli
100g porridge oats
1 handful of sultanas
300ml orange juice
2 eating apples
1 teaspoon of honey (optional)
chopped nuts (optional)

This serves about three. The night before, put the porridge oats, sultanas and orange juice in a bowl, stir, cover and leave overnight. Grate the apples in the morning and stir them straight into the muesli; serve. If you wish, you could add a teaspoon of honey and a few chopped nuts or sultanas in the morning, too, but be careful about quantities. *(Many mueslis are stuffed with dried fruit and nuts at the expense of oats. While these may be tasty, they add lots of calories. This one also needs no milk.)*

Porridge
30g dry porridge oats
chopped dried fruit or fresh fruit (optional)
yoghurt (optional)
honey (optional)
salt (optional)

A bowl of porridge first thing will stand you in good stead during the morning. Per person, you need about 30g dry porridge oats. Put them in a pan and cover well with water; set the pan on a medium heat to simmer and go and do something else for about 5–10 minutes; check the pan occasionally at first to make sure it's not in danger of boiling over or catching, and that the porridge is cooking. Once ready, serve immediately.

You can add some chopped, dried fruit to the oats before cooking, or stir some fresh fruit in afterwards; you can serve porridge with some yoghurt or a teaspoon of honey drizzled on the top; you can even be authentically Scottish and cook it with a pinch of salt if you wish. Try not to use milk instead of the water, but make it skimmed milk if you do. *(Not made with full-cream milk or 'quick' porridge oats.)*

Bread

Steer clear of white bread, and watch out for brown – that's usually white with added colourant. When you're trying to lose weight you want the bread you eat to be as satisfying as possible, so go for whole-meal. And don't bother with 'slimming' breads – think sustainable as well as whether they taste any good (slimming ones usually don't).

You may never have made bread at home, thinking that it might be too fiddly, but you should consider doing so at least some of the time. There are several reasons. Check out the ingredients on an ordinary commercial loaf: do you really need all those E-numbers or that caramelised sugar? Then there's the theory that one of the reasons why so many people seem to have a problem with wheat isn't the wheat as such, but more the added extras that go into commercial loaves and ordinary flour.

If you make your own, you are in control. Nor does baking your own bread have to take for ever; that's a misconception. You mix it, you knead it, you walk away; you don't even have to make a mess. You might go back and knead it again, but then you walk away again. Thirty minutes tops. And it freezes beautifully. You don't need to stop eating bread when you are trying to lose weight; if you eat a lot, though, you should cut down so that those calories can be put towards your overall diet. Try having bread as part of your dish rather than an accompaniment or an extra.

Organic wholemeal bread

500g organic wholemeal bread (or strong) flour
150g organic white bread (or strong) flour
2 level teaspoons of salt
1 level teaspoon of sugar
2 teaspoons of easy-blend yeast or 1 7g sachet
1 tablespoon of olive oil
425ml tepid water

Weigh out the wholemeal and white bread flours. Put them in a large mixing bowl. Add the salt, sugar and yeast. Stir together and add the olive oil; mix once more. Then add the tepid water – one third hot, two-thirds cold – and stir everything; the dough will begin to stick together. Set a timer for 10 minutes. Get your hands into the bowl and begin to knead the dough, turning it and really working it with your hands. After about 5 minutes the texture will begin to change; carry on until the dough gets really elastic – and your timer goes off. Lightly oil two 500g baking tins and sprinkle flour inside. Divide the dough evenly in half and form each portion into a rectangular loaf shape. Place in the tins, cover and leave somewhere warm for 30 minutes. Preheat the oven to 230°C/gas mark 8. By now the dough should be roughly double in size. Pop the tins in the hot oven and cook for 30–35 minutes; you may need to put some foil over them to prevent the tops from catching after about 5 minutes, depending on your oven. The loaves are done when you turn them out of the tins and their bottoms sound hollow if you rap on them. Cool on a rack and slice when cold.
(Contains none of the mysterious ingredients found in most commercial bread; high in fibre.)

Mushrooms on toast

2 small slices of wholemeal or sourdough bread
half a red onion
1 clove of garlic
250g mushrooms .
1 teaspoon of olive oil

dried herbes de Provence or fresh thyme
juice of half a lemon
a sprinkling of paprika

For one person, put two small slices of wholemeal bread or sourdough (if you have any) in the toaster. Chop the red onion, the clove of garlic and as many mushrooms as you want (250g is fine for one; they'll cook down) and heat the olive oil in a large frying pan. Add the onion and cook for a few moments, then add the garlic and mushrooms. Sprinkle over some dried herbes de Provence or some fresh thyme and cook over a medium heat, stirring. The mushrooms will begin to exude their liquid; at this stage, add the lemon juice and paprika. Cook the mushrooms until they are well done, and serve on top of the toast. This is also lovely with a green salad for lunch or dinner.
(Doesn't use any cream; uses very little oil – and no need to butter the toast.)

Eggs

You do not need to avoid eggs; in fact, you should not do so (unless you have been told to for medical reasons). They provide an amazing amount and variety of nutrients for comparatively few calories, and the cholesterol they contain will not harm your health. What does make a difference is how they are cooked. Boiled or poached eggs are usually cooked without anything else, perhaps with a tiny scrape of butter if using a poaching pan. When frying or scrambling eggs, always use a non-stick pan and the minimum amount of butter or, preferably for fried eggs at least, olive oil. Organic eggs have higher nutritional levels, so go for those if you can.

Scrambled eggs with smoked salmon
1–2 slices smoked salmon
2–4 eggs
knob of butter
black pepper

For each person, place a slice or two of smoked salmon on a plate. Break two eggs into a bowl and whisk them well. Warm a tiny knob of butter in a non-stick saucepan until it is foaming, and then tip in the eggs. Stir them well, taking the spoon into the edge of the pan and keeping the egg mixture moving. It will suddenly begin to solidify; remove it from the heat but keep stirring as it will continue to cook in the hot pan. When it is just solid – but not at all leathery – put a generous helping on each plate, and grind some black pepper over the top. Serve immediately. *(Uses very little butter and no milk, which appears in some versions.)*

Lunch, dinner and savoury snacks

Remember to eat regularly and don't be tempted to miss out on lunch just because you're busy. Keep tabs on your choices, portion control and cooking methods, and you should have no real problems – and do remember you can eat as many vegetables as you want with few exceptions (that generally means potatoes), providing they are cooked in the best way – not deep-fried, for instance, and not covered in dressing. There are also a few other things to consider.

Many of us find that we have to eat lunch away from home, whether that means a bought sandwich, a packed lunch or relying on company facilities. The best option, if you are in this position, is the packed lunch – you control the ingredients. A good option is soup, and there is evidence that it can really help to fill you up and stop you feeling hungry for quite some time, so invest in a wide-mouthed flask and take healthy home-made soup for your lunch.

Pastry can be a temptation. Regrettably, perhaps, there's only one thing to do with it if you're trying to lose weight and that's to avoid it as much as possible. You could make it an occasional treat but do bear in mind that pastry is enormously high in calories and usually in saturated fat. Ready-made pies and quiches are also often high in other undesirable ingredients, so if you love a slice of quiche Lorraine every so often, it's worth doing your own pastry or even buying a prepared case and making your own filling. One tip which can help is never to choose a pie with pastry both top and bottom. If you have no choice, leave the pastry lid.

When it comes to salad dressings, invest in a small bottle with a spout and use it to drizzle a little olive oil over a salad most of the time, rather than always making an oil-based dressing and pouring a lot on.

Beans and pulses

It is quite easy to ignore beans and pulses, or to think only of tinned baked beans. But they are a fantastic all-round addition to the diet, providing lots of nutrients including B vitamins and protein, as well as fibre. They are a mainstay of GI diets because they are digested slowly, keeping you feeling full for longer, while also providing a great nutritional punch. Different canned beans are widely available, and dried ones are easy to use – they just need a little planning as they have to be soaked overnight. Both canned and soaked, dried beans should be rinsed well before use, and cooked in fresh water in the case of dried beans; this should help to eliminate any problems with excess wind. In addition, some dried beans should be boiled for the first ten minutes of cooking. The fresher the dried bean, the less time it will take to cook. Lentils are one of the most useful foods in this category, as they do not need overnight soaking. Just rinse and cook in fresh water for about 30 minutes, removing any scum that rises. All beans and pulses are great to add to casseroles and soups, as well as to serve in more specific dishes. It is a shame to confine yourself to tinned baked beans when a broader range of beans and pulses can make such a great contribution to the diet, help weight loss – and taste great.

Butter bean soup with harissa
400g tin of butter beans
half a medium onion
a few small potatoes, unpeeled (about 75g)
half a teaspoon of olive oil
about 500ml stock or water
harissa, to taste

Serves two to three and freezes well. Open, drain and rinse the butter beans; chop the onion and potatoes. Put the olive oil in a pan, add the onion and heat to soften; add the beans and potatoes. Give them a good stir and then add stock or water. Cook until the potatoes are soft, allow to cool and then whizz the soup in a blender until smooth(ish); add more liquid if you wish, but keep it relatively thick. Then add a little harissa – North African chilli and spice paste, widely available – to taste and reheat gently. If you allow the soup to cool before reheating, don't be tempted into adding more liquid; it thickens when cold.
(Uses much less oil than a standard version.)

Hummus

125g dried chickpeas
1 fat clove of garlic, chopped
juice of a lemon
1.5 tablespoons of tahini
half a teaspoon of olive oil

Soak the chickpeas overnight, then rinse and boil for 30 minutes or so (you could also use tinned). Drain the chickpeas, retaining some of their cooking liquid, and put them into a food processor or blender. Add the garlic, lemon juice and tahini; then add a couple of tablespoons of the cooking liquid and the olive oil. Process the chickpea mixture well until smooth and soft, adding more cooking liquid if you need it. Don't make it too sloppy; you should be able to scoop it up with strips of raw vegetables.
(Uses less tahini and olive oil than most recipes.)

Dairy products

Many dairy products are very high in calories, so they need to be approached with a degree of caution. However, they should not be avoided altogether except in exceptional circumstances such as veganism or lactose intolerance, as they are also the best source of calcium. Go for low-fat products – but be wary (see page 62) and check the labels for alternative ingredients. Use yoghurt instead of cream, skimmed instead of full-fat milk and measure quantities of things like cheese carefully. In all these cases, you can make the change gradual rather than sudden.

Cacik
half a large cucumber
150–200g low-fat or no-fat Greek yoghurt
2 crushed cloves of garlic
a large handful of chopped fresh mint
paprika
black pepper

This Turkish salad is similar to the Greek tsatsiki. Use it as a dip for crudités or serve with a wholemeal pitta; these quantities serve two. Chop up the cucumber and, if it is very wet, let it drain in a sieve. Mix the Greek yoghurt with the garlic and add the cucumber. Then mix in the fresh mint. Sprinkle with paprika and black pepper, and serve.
(Uses low- or no-fat yoghurt, and no olive oil.)

Feta, watermelon and pumpkin seed salad
1 tablespoon of pumpkin seeds
1 big slice of watermelon
250g pack of feta
fresh herbs, such as oregano, parsley
salad leaves, to serve

Cheese often goes well in salads, and you don't need much. This serves two. Put the pumpkin seeds in a dry frying pan and toast them until they begin to change colour; remove them from the heat. Cut the watermelon, pick out the seeds and chop the flesh into a bowl. Crumble the feta into the bowl and add the fresh herbs – oregano is good, but parsley works fine. Mix well; serve on a bed of salad leaves and scatter with the toasted pumpkin seeds.
(Does not need a dressing, and uses a comparatively low-calorie cheese.)

Fish and seafood

Go for it when it comes to fish, especially oily fish which is such a great source of omega-3 fats (see page 57). Fish and shellfish are fantastic sources of vitamins and protein, as well, but do think about how they are cooked – deep-fried in batter is not the best choice, and bread-crumbs are worth avoiding too.

Mackerel baked in foil

2 whole mackerel, gutted (without their heads if you prefer)
salt and black pepper
1 slice of lemon
4 sprigs of fresh rosemary
2 cloves of garlic
1 red onion, sliced
2 tablespoons of apple juice or cider

This recipe is easy, delicious *and* good for you – and serves two. Preheat the oven to 200°C/gas mark 6. Rinse the fish and place each one on a large piece of foil. Season them inside and out with salt and black pepper. Put half a slice of lemon inside each fish, then add a couple of sprigs of fresh rosemary to each cavity too. Slice the garlic cloves and add that as well. Scatter each fish with slices of red onion and any excess herbs, and pull the foil up around them. Pour the apple juice or cider over each mackerel and close the foil above it, folding the sides together well to make a sealed parcel. Bake the fish for 25 minutes; serve with a green salad.

(No high-calorie ingredients, no frying, and mackerel is naturally high in the most beneficial oils.)

Prawn tapas

200g of shelled king prawns
2 large cloves of garlic
1 teaspoon of olive oil
juice of a lemon
half a teaspoon of sweet Spanish paprika or a small pinch of ordinary
paprika

The quantity of these garlicky, lemony prawns can be expanded to make
a more substantial dish if you wish; this is a starter or a light meal (with
a green salad) for two, or a main meal for one. Rinse the king prawns
and drain them well. Chop the garlic cloves. Heat the olive oil in a large
frying pan and add the garlic; cook briefly and then tip in the prawns.
Add the lemon juice and the paprika. Stir everything together over a
high heat until the liquid has almost vanished. Serve immediately.
(Uses very little oil.)

Salade Niçoise

1 egg per person
a bed of lettuce leaves
some chopped ripe tomatoes
a few rings of red onion
some chopped pepper
cucumber rings
chopped black olives
small tin of anchovies
tin of tuna in spring water
olive oil
balsamic vinegar

Hard-boil an egg per person. Arrange the lettuce leaves, tomatoes, red
onion, pepper and cucumber rings on each plate – whatever you want,
but don't add anything cooked. Scatter some chopped black olives over.
Drain the oil from the anchovies and blot them well on kitchen paper
to remove the excess; arrange a few on each plate. Then drain the tuna

(the tin size depends on how many servings) and flake the fish over the salad. Shell the eggs, cut into quarters and put four quarters on each plate. Drizzle with olive oil and balsamic vinegar. Serve immediately. *(No potatoes; tuna in spring water – or you could use one in brine, well rinsed – rather than oil; blotted anchovies: all lower the calorie count.)*

Meat and poultry

It is worth being cautious when it comes to meat. Red meat, in general, should be restricted or reduced in quantity, and not just because of the effect it can have on your weight, but also because it is high in saturated fat. So cut it back, and always trim off excessive fat before cooking or buy less fatty alternatives, like lean lamb mince rather than normal minced beef. Poultry skin is also high in saturated fat, so remove that before cooking, whenever practical. There are also some cuts which are better for you than others because they are lower in fat. Pork, for example, is often considered fatty, but think about pork fillet, sometimes called tenderloin – it is actually lower in fat (and in calories) than many other cuts, or other meats. Strips of pork fillet can be a lovely addition to a stir-fry. Another useful approach is to cut quantities in something like a stew or casserole, adding other ingredients – more vegetables or pulses – instead. Cooking methods can make a real difference, so be careful and don't do anything where you have to add lots of extra fat.

Chicken kebabs
2 skinless chicken breasts
2 or 3 red onions
1 large green pepper
1 tablespoon of olive oil
juice of a lemon
a crushed clove of garlic
some chopped fresh herbs (especially rosemary)

For four generous skewers, chop the chicken breasts into cubes. Then chop the red onions and green pepper. Mix together the olive oil, lemon juice, garlic and some chopped fresh herbs – rosemary is delicious. Put this marinade mixture in a sealable plastic bag (without holes!) and add the chicken and vegetables. Close the bag and ensure everything is mixed together; put it in the fridge for 30 minutes. If you are using wooden skewers, put them in water to soak. Then assemble the kebabs, alternating the different ingredients. Brush them with the remaining marinade and cook over a barbecue or under a grill until ready – turn them regularly. Test the chicken to make sure it is cooked before serving; it shouldn't be pink in the middle.

(Uses comparatively little oil in the marinade, but it coats the meat and vegetables well because of the bag technique – the amount could even be reduced further if wished. No skin on the chicken.)

Lemon and herb roast chicken
1 chicken
1 lemon
olive oil
dried herbes de Provence

Preheat the oven to 200°C/gas mark 6. Use a roasting tin with a rack, and put the chicken on the rack. Cut the lemon in quarters and put three of the pieces inside the bird. Pour a little olive oil on to your hand and rub it over the outside of the chicken, then squeeze the last lemon quarter over it and add that to the other pieces inside. Sprinkle the chicken lavishly with dried herbes de Provence and put it in the oven. Roast for 20 minutes per 500g weight, plus 30 minutes. After it has been in the oven for about 20–25 minutes, cover it with foil. When time is up, check that it is done by sticking a knife into the flesh; if the juices run clear, it's fine. Set the bird to one side to rest for 10 minutes before carving, keeping it covered with the foil. Don't make gravy with the fatty juices (unless it is for other people) and don't eat the skin. How many this serves depends on how big your chicken is.

(By cooking the chicken on a rack, the fat drains away and the bird doesn't sit in it; the foil helps to keep it moist, so it doesn't need to be basted with the hot fat, either.)

Nuts and seeds

Both nuts and seeds are high in calories, but they are also high in nutrients; just two Brazil nuts, for instance, will supply your entire daily requirement of selenium. So don't cut them out (though salted ones should be restricted) but be careful instead. A few nuts or seeds, or a few of both, can make a great topping or addition to salads and breakfast cereals – and they are delicious lightly toasted in a dry frying pan and scattered on top of low-calorie Greek yoghurt.

Toasted seed and nut coleslaw
3 or 4 walnuts
1 tablespoon pumpkin seeds
1 tablespoon of sunflower seeds
about 150g of green or white cabbage
2 large carrots
some chopped red onion (optional)
80ml of low-fat yoghurt
1 teaspoon of Dijon mustard

This makes enough for two substantial helpings; it will keep in the fridge for several days but prepare the nuts and seeds just before you serve it.

Chop the walnuts. In a dry frying pan, toast the nuts with the pumpkin and sunflower seeds; when they begin to smell toasted and pop, remove the pan from the heat and put the seeds and nuts on a plate. Shred the cabbage and grate the carrots; add some chopped red onion if you like it. Mix them together in a large bowl. In another bowl mix the low-fat yoghurt with the Dijon mustard, then add this to the coleslaw and stir everything together well – do not be tempted to add more yoghurt unless it looks really dry, but carry on stirring until the coating is even. Spoon on to plates and top with a handful of the toasted seeds and walnuts.

(Doesn't incorporate lots of high-calorie ingredients, such as mayonnaise; restricts the quantity of nuts.)

Pasta and rice

Pasta and rice are typical of those foods which you will need to measure at first, though you may eventually find that four medium handfuls of penne, for instance, is near enough to 100g for you to be able to use it as a shortcut. Overdoing it can make quite a difference.

When it comes to pasta sauces, be very cautious if you are eating out as they are often also high in calories. Ready-made ones – well, avoid them if you can. It's not only the calories (though some are acceptable, almost), it's the other unhealthy additives as well. Pasta sauces are easy to make, taking next to no time in most cases. Wholemeal pastas are also worth investigating, particularly if your only experience of them is being force-fed something claggy in the 1970s or 80s. They have changed a lot, and the best brands are not remotely heavy, plus they stand up to really punchy sauces much better than white pastas. They're also, of course, better for you in GI terms.

Sicilian spaghetti sauce
2 400g tins of chopped tomatoes
2 chopped cloves of garlic
1 anchovy fillet
1 green pepper
2 tablespoons of drained capers

This freezes beautifully, so save any excess; the quantities here are enough for four generous helpings. Open the chopped tomatoes and put them in a large pan. Add the garlic and cook over a low heat for 30 minutes. Blot the anchovy fillet on kitchen paper and chop it into small pieces; add it to the pan too. Chop a green pepper into small pieces and add that, together with the drained capers. Leave the sauce to cook gently for at least another 30 minutes; check to make sure it isn't catching and give it a stir every so often.

(No oil needed in the sauce, anchovy fillet blotted to remove any excess – and no Parmesan needed for serving, which is also true for most tomato-based sauces.)

Stir-fried vegetables with rice and egg

40g basmati rice per person

mixed vegetables, e.g. 1 red pepper, 2 carrots, a couple of bunches of spring onions, rings of red onion, slices of courgette, strips of cucumber

2 cloves of garlic

2cm cube of fresh ginger

chopped chilli (optional)

1 teaspoon of sesame oil

1 egg

soy sauce, tamari for preference

Stir-fries are fantastic for anyone trying to lose weight. Cook 40g basmati rice per person and drain. Finely chop a variety of vegetables while the rice is cooking – whatever you have to hand, as long as there's plenty. Chop the garlic and ginger; add some chopped chilli if you wish. Heat the sesame oil in a large non-stick wok and, when it is really hot, add the garlic, ginger and chilli, if using. Let them cook briefly, and then add whichever vegetables need the longest cooking – in the list above, that would be the carrots and pepper. Let them cook for few minutes, then add the rest. Stir frequently. Break the egg into a small container and stir it up (with a chopstick, if possible). By now the vegetables should be cooking nicely; they should still be crunchy. Add the cooked rice to the wok and stir well, then add a splash of soy sauce. Clear a space in the centre of the wok and pour in the egg; stir it frantically with the chopstick at first, as it begins to set, then mix it into the rest of the stir-fry – and serve.

(Oil is kept to a minimum; lots of vegetables instead of lots of rice.)

Vegetables

Vegetables are one area where you can pile your plate high without too much trouble, providing you remember one or two guidelines. The first is that the 'pile it high' permission does not apply to potatoes and any other starchy vegetables; treat them as you would rice or pasta when considering portions (see page 66) and keep quantities to a minimum.

Potatoes, in fact, are 'banned' on some GI diets, except when they are baked in their skins; sweet potatoes are used as a substitute.

The second guideline is to bear in mind how vegetables are cooked – an Indian vegetarian curry may well contain lots of vegetables, but it probably also contains lots of ghee (clarified butter) or oil, and maybe something high in calories like coconut. Watch vegetables which are often served with butter and either cut it out or reduce it dramatically; similarly, creamy sauces are not a good idea to include on anything other than an infrequent basis. Don't eat any vegetables covered in batter and be cautious about anything fried. To maximise the benefits from vegetables, eat as wide a variety as you can (see pages 55–6).

Aubergine curry with tomato raita
2 teaspoons of oil
1 medium aubergine (about 400g)
1 medium onion
3 tablespoons of tomato purée
a pinch of salt
1 teaspoon of paprika
1 fresh chilli
a pinch of garam masala
For the raita:
2 small tomatoes
100g of low-fat yoghurt

This healthy dry curry serves two. Heat the oil in a large non-stick pan with a lid. Chop the aubergine and finely slice the onion. Put the tomato purée in a mug and mix it with a little warm water. Cook the onion in the pan until soft, then add the salt and paprika; stir. Add the aubergine and the tomato purée, and mix to combine everything and to ensure the aubergines do not stick; you can add more water if necessary. Chop the fresh chilli, being careful not to rub your eyes, and add that to the pan – you can use more or less, to taste. Cover the pan and lower the heat to a gentle simmer for another 5 minutes, and add a pinch of garam masala. Cook for a further 10–15 minutes until the aubergines are soft, and serve. There shouldn't be a lot of sauce, but this curry can be accompanied with a tomato raita. To make the raita, remove the seeds from the tomatoes, and add the flesh to the yoghurt, stirring well.

(Uses much less oil than conventional curry recipes.)

Ribollita

2 medium onions
4 large carrots
2 cloves of garlic
1 teaspoon of olive oil
400g tin of chopped tomatoes
400g tin of borlotti beans
1 cavolo nero (or Savoy cabbage)

A traditional Italian soup, packed with healthy ingredients, which serves three to four – and freezes very well. Chop the onions, carrots and garlic. Put the olive oil in a large pan and cook the vegetables for about 10 minutes over a low-to-medium heat, stirring to ensure they don't catch. Drain the chopped tomatoes (save the juice for a pasta sauce, perhaps), and put them in the pan. Continue cooking for 30 minutes. Drain and rinse the borlotti beans. Chop up plenty of cavolo nero (or Savoy cabbage) and add it, together with the beans and enough water to cover the vegetables. Simmer for another 30 minutes and serve. You can, if you wish, put half the beans in the soup and mash the other half, adding them just before serving to warm through. The soup should be thick.

(Many versions of ribollita include bread to thicken the soup, and lots more olive oil.)

Puddings and sweet things

There's no reason to stop eating sweet things when you are dieting but it is one area where it is vital to keep the M word – moderation – in mind. You may, however, need to avoid cakes; it is almost impossible to make these in such a way that they can form part of a weight-loss effort. It is better, therefore, to confine yourself to a slice of cake as a very occasional treat, and to steer clear of gateaux piled high with cream or cakes covered in icing. If you stick to plain(ish) cakes, and only eat them occasionally, you should be fine. It is, however, one of the first areas to look at if you do have a sweet tooth and don't seem to be lowering your weight. Pastry is another danger area, as it is high in both saturated fat and calories, and sweet pies are often also high in sugar. If you have no choice, you can always leave all or some of the pastry.

By and large, base desserts on fruit, and be sensible about what other things you use – watch out, for example, for accompaniments like cream, ice cream and custard; low-fat Greek yoghurt can make a good substitute. A piece of perfect fresh fruit can, however, be an equally great way to end a meal. When it comes to fruit salads, there's no need to have a sugary syrup as a base: use a little alcohol instead. Just one tablespoon of peach schnapps lifts a summer fruit salad out of the ordinary; Cointreau goes well with anything involving oranges or citrus, and kirsch is fab with berries.

Fruit

Fruits are packed with minerals, vitamins, fibre – eat the skins whenever possible – and antioxidants, which play a powerfully protective role in the body. Have at least one piece of fresh fruit every day, using it as a substitute for a less healthy snack, and do try and go for the whole fruit rather than juice. Fresh is best, though it should be washed; go for organic citrus fruit if you can as the skins can absorb pesticides. Frozen is often OK (particularly in winter) and tinned is disappointingly low in the best nutrients and high in sugar by comparison. Dried fruit is excellent nutritionally, but can be high in calories so measure quantities in the beginning at least, and try and find unsulphured versions.

Bananas with rum and cinnamon
bananas, 1 per person
a little white rum

cinnamon
soft brown sugar (optional)

These are perfect for a barbecue, but can be easily baked, cooked under a hot grill or on a ridged pan. Allow one large banana per person, and wrap it well in foil – do not peel. Place the banana parcels on the barbecue and cook, turning over at least once, until you can feel them soften. Unwrap the parcels on to a plate, slit the banana skin along its length and pour in a little white rum; sprinkle with cinnamon and – if you wish – a small amount of soft brown sugar. Eat!
(No need for cream and no frying.)

Iced berries
1 cup of strawberries
1 cup of blueberries
1 cup of raspberries
6 ice cubes
2 teaspoons of kirsch

Chop the strawberries and place them in a large bowl. Add the blueberries and raspberries and stir them together. Put the ice cubes in a blender together with a tablespoon of water, and process until the cubes have been crushed. Tip them into the bowl with the berries and mix everything together quickly. Spoon into serving dishes, drizzle a teaspoon of kirsch over each one and serve immediately. This is an adaptable recipe; you can use as much fruit as you wish (though you would need more ice; this would do for two).
(You don't need ice cream for a refreshing cold treat on a hot day.)

Sugar, sweets and chocolate

Yes … or rather, no. There are many ways of satisfying a sweet tooth besides eating the often nutritionally bad choices available all over the place, and there is some evidence that the taste for sugar is addictive. This is one taste addiction which it is worth trying to break as it can have such an immediate impact on both your weight and your health. Whatever you do, make sure any sugary things you eat provide more than empty calories and go easy anyway.

There is a ray of light for the sweet-toothed, though – chocolate isn't all bad. Choose varieties with a high cocoa content, 70 per cent or over, eat small quantities slowly and really savour it. The better the chocolate, the more there is to enjoy in the taste, and the more satisfying it is (providing, of course, you don't just wolf it down). This is one area where concentrating on what you are eating can make a real difference and, when you do, a 10g square is likely to be enough.

Chocolate cherries
1 cup of cherries
50g dark chocolate (70 per cent cocoa solids or above)

Select and wash some perfect cherries, leaving the stalks on; don't use any with blemishes and dry them on a tea towel. Line a baking tray with greaseproof paper. Put a bowl over a pan of boiling water – don't let the bowl touch the water itself – and break the dark chocolate into the bowl in small pieces. Stir the chocolate chunks carefully, and when they have all melted remove the bowl from the pan. Dip the cherries partly into the melted chocolate, holding them by the stalk, and put them on the baking tray. When all the chocolate is used up, put the baking tray in the fridge for at least an hour. Other fruits can be used in the same way – strawberries work well.
(Good chocolate, and not too much of it ...)

Dried fruit sweets
a few hazelnuts
2 tablespoons of sunflower seeds
2 tablespoons of pumpkin seeds
sesame seeds (optional)
250g of mixed dried fruit – sultanas, apricots, raisins, a few cranberries
2–3 tablespoons of orange juice
a grind of nutmeg

half a teaspoon of cinnamon
ground nuts or coconut, for coating

Grind the hazelnuts with the sunflower and pumpkin seeds; add some sesame seeds if you have them to hand. Put the ground nuts and seed mix in a food processor with the mixed dried fruit and a couple of tablespoons of orange juice. Process them briefly and add a little more juice if the mixture seems very stiff. Then add the nutmeg and cinnamon and process again. Transfer the sticky mixture into a bowl. Put the ground nuts or coconut in another bowl. Form the dried fruit mix into small balls, rolling them between your hands, and then roll them in the ground nuts or coconut. Shake off any excess and put the finished sweets, one by one, on a plate. When all are done, chill in the fridge for an hour. They will keep for a week.

(Not that low in calories, of course, so be careful – but much healthier than a box of chocolates.)

A note on ready-made food

It is easy to condemn all processed food, but if you are truly puritanical about it, you would find that your diet was not particularly sustainable. There are some things which are just more convenient to buy than make – but that doesn't include complete meals or things like cook-in sauces, as the apparent convenience and time saving involved are hugely outweighed by the health benefits of making your own and controlling the ingredients.

Ready-made food fits into one of three categories: the good, the bad (that's most of it, in reality and in one way or another) and the inevitable. Into the good, or at least really useful, category come spice pastes such as harissa and bottled mayonnaise, which you are unlikely to make from scratch every time you need a spoonful – though you could, in theory at least, do so comparatively easily. However, do watch the calories in bought mayo specifically, and in other bought substitutes for things you could possibly make, such as jam or marmalade. The low-calorie versions are often the ones with the highest number of artificial ingredients, so you may have to do some balancing here, as well as some careful measuring. Tinned baked beans probably fall into the 'good' group, too; though making your own is easy, it does take a bit of planning and baked beans on toast is likely to be an impulse meal. Read the labels on all your store-cupboard favourites and check your assumptions carefully because high-calorie options can easily sneak in.

The bad ones we all know about, in our hearts. They can be high in calories, high in artificial ingredients, high in fats (and the wrong sort of fats), high in salt, high in sugar and may include that high-fructose corn syrup ... Ready meals, biscuits, fizzy drinks, high-fat salty snacks, sugary breakfast cereals, almost anything which has been through a lot of processing is worth avoiding. If you find yourself hovering over something in the supermarket which you suspect falls into this category, check the ingredients. If you don't recognise any of them, put it back. If there are lots of them, put it back. And if there's anything you recognise but wouldn't expect to find – lots of salt in something ostensibly sweet, perhaps – put it back. All of these are signs of something that is highly processed, and that's what you want to avoid. Also beware of slogans like 'healthy' or 'diet', because nine times out of ten that's all they are – slogans. It is also worth noting that many processed foods, even the old favourites, are actually worse now than they used to be in terms of sugar, fat and calorie content, which has often come about as manufacturers have changed the recipes to compensate for the lack of taste as they reduced salt levels.

There's a bit of blurring between the 'inevitable' category and the 'good' one, but the inevitables include things like tomato ketchup or Marmite which it would be almost impossible to replicate at home. You couldn't recreate Marmite unless you happened to live in a brewery, it does have wonderful levels of B vitamins, and although it is salty, you use so little that you can afford it. Go easy with these 'inevitables' and keep them to a minimum. They are often high in calories too, so measure or weigh unless you know you'll use very little (that's Marmite again) – and, once more, check your assumptions; there is no way in which chocolate biscuits are 'inevitable', not *really*. Nor are they 'good'.

Finally, bear in mind that you can often make passable alternatives to some of the apparent inevitables at home. Commercial tomato soup is one – a tomato and red pepper soup, made with some fresh thyme, thickened with a few small potatoes and then liquidised, is quick to make. Not only is it a good alternative in terms of taste, it's also lower in salt, and minus the sugar and artificial preservatives in the commercial versions. Freshly made apple purée is a great alternative to a bottled apple sauce, and you could add fresh berries to low-fat natural yoghurt as an alternative to the (often high in sugar) low-fat fruit yoghurts. With time, you'll be able to come up with alternatives to most of your own current choices. It really is worth doing.

8 Getting fit – formal exercise and the alternatives

Exercise really is good for your health (though do be careful, and consult your doctor if you are overweight and have not taken any exercise for some time), but you do have to be realistic and not expect too much from it when it comes to actually reducing your waistline.

Don't be put off by the idea of exercise, either. Never assume that exercise has to be done in a formal setting, with an instructor shouting at you, or in the company of other sweaty individuals. Think laterally because there are lots of options, and there will undoubtedly be something that suits you and which enables you to include more activity in your life. It could be something like dancing, energetic dog walking or clearing overgrown paths; you don't have to run or go to the gym. And one of the best forms of exercise is so obvious that most of us hardly think of it as 'exercise' as such: walking. It's also one of the easiest forms of exercise to increase, and that in turn helps to increase the overall amount of exercise you take.

Exercise *can* improve your overall sense of wellbeing, reduce your blood pressure and even reduce your risk of cancer, so it can help you live longer. What it probably will *not* do, and this has been borne out by a number of large and wide-ranging studies, is bring clear benefits in terms of weight loss; it's part of the solution, rather than a solution in itself. One of the problems with exercise is that the more energy your body uses, the more it requires – and that tends to come in the form of increased calorie intake rather than increased use of existing fat stores. The fact that exercise probably won't bring about a dramatic decrease in weight as such doesn't mean you can afford to ignore it, however. There are so many other health benefits which exercise can definitely bring that you should go for it. Exercise does seem to have an impact, however, when it comes to maintaining weight loss – with some provisos – and there is evidence that those dieters who lose weight and then succeed in keeping it off are the ones who have managed to integrate more exercise into their life. Bear in mind that the more muscle you have, the more it will help to boost your basal metabolic rate – muscle uses more calories than fat, even when you are doing nothing – which is what you want to happen.

Keep your expectations realistic when it comes to practical considerations, too. If the nearest bellydancing class involves a long journey, then you're probably not going to persist; see if the much closer salsa class can't satisfy your urge to shake your body about. If your energy levels are really low in the evenings, exercise at lunchtime instead. And if something really appeals to you, however ordinary or extraordinary it is, you'll find making the commitment easier – so if you have always genuinely wanted to bellydance, give it a go anyway. The other thing to do is not restrict yourself to one activity, once you get a taste for it, but try something else as well. If you find the thought of team games or exercise classes makes your blood run cold, then there are plenty of other options available, and exercise doesn't have to be alarming. In fact, it should be anything but alarming if you're going to carry on with it. Here are some suggestions for adding more activity to your life.

Formal exercise

There are so many different forms of exercise to choose from, it's worth doing some investigating. Ask around; many people are already doing something they love and are quite happy to tell you about it; they may also be able to recommend particular classes or instructors. It is almost inevitable that you'll find something you can enjoy.

Time to examine various possibilities, to look at what they can do for you, and see how you can make them part of your everyday life. The specific examples below have been selected because they are particularly easy to incorporate into your life almost automatically. And automatic is what they need to become, because the more you do, the more you'll enjoy it, and the more you enjoy it, the more you'll keep doing it. That's important, because some experts have demonstrated that intermittent exercise – yo-yo exercise, perhaps – can actually make you feel worse. If you can find a form of exercise which you really like you are much less likely to fall into this trap, so do some testing to get it right – and then have fun.

Cycling

Like other forms of exercise, cycling needs to be done regularly; simply getting the bike out once in a while will not make a lot of difference. On a regular basis, moderate cycling is good, but cycling up hills and fast cycling is even better, and has even been described as doing an aerobics class sitting down (the professionals, incidentally, say that the best way to cycle up a hill is not to attack it like a maniac). You get a good cardiovascular workout and can build lower-body muscle. However, you do need to ensure that you are safe, and that doesn't just mean from motorists; you need to make sure that you don't put too much strain on your heart or joints. As with everything, build up gently. Take reasonable road-safety precautions when you're cycling, and always wear sensible shoes and a good protective helmet. You may feel like a fool, but it could save your life. Make sure your lights work, too!

Exercise classes

Many people, particularly those who are overweight, find the prospect of an exercise class daunting. There's no need, though; most of the people in a class will be too busy concentrating on themselves and their own moves to worry about anyone else.

Check out alternatives, as there is a wide variety of classes around, from aerobics to yoga and from core training to kick boxing and capoeira, the Brazilian martial art. They tend to change too, as new disciplines become popular and interest in older ones falls away. Bear in mind that all classes are different, even within a specific discipline, and it may be possible for you to try a single one as a taster to see if it suits you – well, principally, if the instructor suits you. You might also be able to sit in on a session. It is also worth exploring the possibility of going with a friend, as that automatically makes the prospect of attending a

Prepare yourself

It's no good taking up exercise if all you do is make yourself physically uncomfortable or hurt yourself so much that you have to give up. Good footwear is essential, and take care when you're buying it. Always try on sports shoes when your feet are at their most swollen – i.e. the largest size that the shoes will need to accommodate when you are using them rather than just trying them on in a shop; it's even worth trying a size larger than normal. Relying on only one pair of walking boots or trainers is a mistake. They need to dry out between sessions, and trainers in particular can get disgusting quickly. It's not just the smell, it's the chance of fungal infection, so take this seriously. Walking boots can be a bit different, so there's more information on choosing them on page 134.

Women should invest in a good sports bra; you could damage your breasts if you undertake an exercise regime in an ordinary one, though this is fine for walking; high-impact exercise – like running or using many of the machines at the gym – has the worst effect. For every mile you run, recent research has shown that your boobs bounce up and down for 135 metres. Do protect them.

Finally, check with your GP if you have not done any exercise for ages, especially if you are very overweight. If you are over the age of 50 this may also be a good idea. Be careful: warm up before starting and wind down afterwards; don't push yourself too far; stop if something hurts rather than pressing on with whatever you are doing; and keep hydrated.

class less daunting; you can also encourage each other, whether you're daunted or not. Nor do you have to join an expensive private gym to participate in a good exercise class; many local authority leisure centres run them and there are also some independent ones undertaken by private instructors (though it might be a good idea to check on their qualifications; they should not object and if they do, regard it as a bad sign). Finally, whatever class you decide to attend, stop if the class is doing something which is too hard for you until it eases up again. Don't push yourself too far, or allow yourself to be pushed too far by the instructor.

Aerobics

This is still popular, and taking a class can be a great way to ensure you get a good cardiovascular workout. Aerobics can, however, also be heavy on the joints, so it is worth asking about a low-impact class, where you will always keep one foot on the ground. Good footwear is absolutely vital in helping to reduce the impact further. You should take this seriously because an injudicious choice of shoes or too many high-impact work-outs can cause stress fractures. One other thing – you might think you'd use up a lot of calories in an aerobics class, but in actual fact you'd be likely to use slightly more playing badminton or tennis, jogging or swimming – or climbing the stairs for the same length of time (unlikely though you'd be to do that, even on a machine at the gym). You'd burn a lot more playing handball too. Appearances can be deceptive when it comes to calories used.

Gym sessions

Many people instantly associate exercise with going to a gym, but don't splash out on a gym membership unless you are already certain that you are going to use it, and that gym-based exercise is the right choice for you. It isn't, for many people; it can be boring for one thing, which is something you won't know until you try. If you're tempted by the thought of running machines rather than walking round the local park, try a local authority gym first and see if you like it, or take advantage of taster sessions and open days.

It can be quite easy to injure yourself at a gym, so it makes sense to be careful. Always do an induction session, even if you think you know what you're doing. Take professional advice as well, and make sure you stick to it. Poor technique is very common, so check some of these frequent mistakes. You can make exercise too easy, for a start; many people who use a stair-climber have the steps too shallow. Gripping the handlebars tightly on a stair-climber will also decrease the workload and add tension; the same applies on an elliptical trainer. Then there's failing to alter settings when you get on a machine someone else has just left. Make sure the seat is the right height on a stationary bike, for instance; if it's too high you'll have to pedal on tiptoe and if it's too low you'll be cramped. It's easy to set the right height: put a heel on one pedal and extend your leg until it's straight. If you find yourself leaning forwards, try not to round your back. But the biggest error that almost everyone makes at some time is the failure to warm up properly. Always, always do this. Cold muscles combined with sudden movement are a potential disaster area. As is not exercising very often and then trying to pack masses of activity into a single session – it puts too much strain on the heart.

Weight training

Working with weights builds muscle through resistance, which can help boost your BMR, and many people find that it helps when maintaining their weight loss. Once again you should find an instructor if you are at all unsure of what you are doing and one of the best places to start is at a gym, though you can do some forms of weight training at home. One of the most important things is to achieve balance; to protect your joints you need to exercise the flexor and extensor muscles around them in relative proportion, and that's why you need an instructor. There is one thing to add – many women are put off weight training because this is all too often seen as the 'boys' area of a gym. Just ignore that and give it a go.

Running and jogging

Running beats almost every other form of exercise when it comes to calorie expenditure (and fast running is the overall winner). Assessing this is frought with variables, but an average man would use 700 calories in an hour spent running at a relatively leisurely, ten-minute mile, pace. It has many benefits in terms of improving cardiovascular health and developing the leg muscles, but the counter to this is the damage which the repeated impact of running can cause. It can stress the spine, as well as the knees and ankles, and the answer is to improve your technique and make sure you are wearing the best possible footwear. Do invest in excellent running shoes, as they can help to reduce the impact on your joints. If you fancy taking up running, then build up slowly – start with walking, progress to walking up a gradient, then jogging and only then move on to running. Also, you should seek advice from someone who knows what they are talking about when it comes to technique; it's not worth the risk of permanent damage and back pain.

There are other things to watch out for, like a tendency to always take the same route or even always run on the same side of the road – if you do always use the same piece of road the camber could cause problems, as one leg will always be hitting the ground at a different level to the other. Variety is good for you. As a final caveat, running can get very competitive, so don't let this stress you out. Instead, try to concentrate on and enjoy the tension-relieving aspects of exercise as a way to wind down after a heavy day at work.

Swimming

Though swimming can provide a good workout for the heart and lungs, it's not the most energetic form of exercise unless you really work at it. It is excellent, however, for anyone with any joint problems or injury as the water provides the necessary support, and it is a good all-round exercise for both flexibility and body strength. It is important that you go to the pool regularly to really benefit from swimming, so try and swim continuously for 30 minutes – count lengths if you want to and increase them over time – at least three times a week. If it's been a long time since you did any swimming, think about having a few one-to-one lessons to improve your technique; breathing rhythms and timing tend to drift a little, for instance. Using a small pool is not so good, but it is better than nothing – ideally you want a pool of at least 25m.

Aquarobics

Like swimming, aquarobics is great for anybody with joint problems. It can also be good for toning muscles as the water exerts resistance in both directions as you move, but classes which are too gentle will not help that much; you still need a workout and the more movement you do in the water, the more your body works. The greatest effect which most people experience with aquarobics is an increased sense of well-being: it's fun, and that really is good for you.

Gentler classes

Swimming, running, cycling and so forth are all forms of cardio-vascular exercise that work by increasing your heart rate so that oxygen is pumped round the body in the bloodstream to take energy to the

Sponsorship

Sponsorship is a great way of ensuring you get your exercise in, whatever the weather and whatever good films are on television. You may have a charity you particularly want to support, so find out if they are organising anything like a fun run and join in; you could rope in friends and colleagues as well – and exercising with friends in aid of a good cause is a great way to spend your time, benefitting both your health and other people. Your colleagues don't actually have to join in, of course – they could just put their hands in their pockets and pay when you succeed.

muscles. Gentler forms of exercise that tone the muscles without making you out of breath are also valuable, and they can help to make you look better by flattening stomachs and firming thighs. Try a few and choose the method that seems to work best for you.

Pilates

A huge number of people have attended a Pilates class at some time, and many find them fantastic. This scheme of exercise was designed by Joseph Pilates to strengthen and lengthen dancers' muscles. Its fans often speak of improved posture and body shape, but there are other benefits as well – though all is dependent on the teacher. (You should check that your Pilates instructor is properly qualified.)

Pilates is often recommended for people who haven't done much exercise, but again this is related to the abilities of the teacher. A good one will be able to show you how to strengthen your muscles gradually and protect any weak areas from injury. The movements are very subtle but focus on building core strength round your middle, which helps to protect the spine (and flatten the tummy). It is also worth asking about the size of a Pilates class, as a large one will not allow the teacher to give the right level of instruction.

Specialist Pilates studios will have equally specialist equipment, but most teaching is now done in ordinary health clubs and gyms. If you have ever done any yoga, you may find some of the stretching exercises in Pilates vaguely similar.

Tai chi

Tai chi looks deceptively gentle, and in some ways it is. It combines slow, relaxed movement with an alert but calm mental state – and it also has considerable health benefits. It really does seem to make you feel good mentally, and full of energy. It also lowers blood pressure and supports the joints as you move without an overly harsh impact; it's been shown to decrease pain significantly, for instance, in people with arthritis. Even better, diabetes sufferers who do tai chi have seen clear benefits – they've reported more consistent blood-sugar levels (which could be linked to the weight loss some have also mentioned) and increased energy. Tai chi is outstanding for improving balance and co-ordination, and seems to have good effects on the health of both the lungs and the heart.

It is important to find a good teacher, though, as tai chi is not something you can teach yourself, so do some investigating if this appeals to you. Because the relationship with the instructor is important, you are often encouraged to meet first. You are also expected to do some practising at home. If you actually enjoy exertion when you exercise, then tai chi is not a good choice for you; it builds strength in other ways. But don't think it will be a doddle, either – it can be extraordinarily difficult.

Yoga

Yoga classes may be the gentlest introduction to the world of group exercise if you've not done any since your school days, and yoga itself is a great form of exercise for almost anyone. Doing yoga regularly will enhance your flexibility, agility and should also increase your strength.

A beginner's class will normally include people of both sexes as well as of almost every age, shape and fitness level, and they are usually very welcoming. Yoga is generally very safe and will help to tone your body, and many women find it helpful during pregnancy, but you do need be realistic and use some discretion in the type of yoga class you attend. In most classes you move into a position, hold it while focusing on your breathing, and then move into another position. Ashtanga yoga is much more athletic, as you spring from one position into another instead. This does not make it ideal for beginners, unless they are already fit, and it is also very dependent on the calibre of the instructors. It is possible to injure yourself doing Ashtanga yoga, which is quite difficult to do with other types, so do be careful. If a friend offers to take you along to a 'wonderful' yoga class to get you started, make sure you check which type is involved. In all kinds of yoga classes, the teacher should keep a close eye on what you are doing and will often come round to correct postures, so make sure that they know of any injury or physical problems you may have. Finally, yoga is a holistic approach to fitness, and aims to provide mental as well as physical benefits.

Lateral thinking

It's easy to fall into the trap of believing that exercise has to be formal, something set to one side in a mental box. Of course, that's not the case, and many people find that box somewhat off-putting anyway.

The key here is making simple activities part of your everyday routine. A good one is to walk more; walk to get the paper rather than getting the car out; collect the kids from school on foot; do some gardening for ten minutes every day. Park the car as far away from the supermarket entrance as you can, rather than jockeying for that tempting spot close to the doors; use stairs instead of lifts and walk – or run – up escalators rather than letting them carry you. Wash the car yourself instead of either taking it to the car wash or bribing any passing children. Do a few simple exercises during ad breaks in television programmes or run on the spot, and 'lose' the remote so you have to get up to reach it. You don't need expensive equipment, either: you can always improvise with something like two 400g tins of tomatoes, used as weights for bicep curls; the bottom step on the stairs for step-ups or a door frame for standing 'press-ups'. If you have children, take them swimming or go to a dance class with one of your friends. It doesn't matter what you do, just do more.

There are even smaller things that you can do to encourage flexibility. Stretch for things; put them just out of reach so that you have to make some effort to get them. If you drop something, stretch down to get it, but keep your legs straight. Make an effort at first and it will become automatic. Try holding your stomach in a little when you get up in the morning, and see how long you can keep that up; it's been described as acting like 'an all-day sit-up' and is also an old French tip for encouraging a flat stomach. It's all about tone.

The trick is to look for little ways in which to adapt extra activity to your particular lifestyle. If you take the bus to work, or commute into central London on the underground, get off a stop before you need to and walk the rest of the way. And standing is better for you than sitting down too, so don't charge into a carriage, pushing people out of the way in your rush for a seat – stand and feel virtuous; after all, the chances are that you'll spend most of the day sitting at work. Take a walk at lunchtime; it will refresh you as well as give you some exercise, and it's always good to get a break from the office. Give it some thought, decide what basic changes you can make without too much pain, and then stick with them. But do be flexible and sensible; there's no point slogging miles through a torrential downpour when you could have made a quick dash for a closer bus stop. Don't make yourself unnecessarily miserable; you'll just give up.

Almost everyone has used the 'I'm just too busy' reason for not exercising. If you find yourself beginning to think along these lines at this point, be hard-nosed about it and test your assumption. Keep a record of how you actually spend your free time during one week. How much went on watching television or fiddling around on the Internet to no good purpose? Most of us do pass some of our time in this way. Can you really not manage to give up a little of this, say 30 minutes twice a week? Here are a few alternatives to classes and team sports that would be a great way to fill any new-found spare time.

Conservation volunteering

There are many possibilities for adding something to your local environment while at the same time getting some exercise, from local initiatives – maybe removing litter from a street or unblocking clogged streams in a park – to more formal schemes. Clearing footpaths is always useful and can be quite high-intensity exercise; in fact, it's one of the things which the British Trust for Conservation Volunteers (or BTCV) uses in its 'green gyms' scheme, where volunteers meet up on a regular basis. These schemes are scattered across the country, so it is worth checking them out and seeing if they might suit you (www2.btcv.org.uk/display/greengym). If there isn't a convenient one, you could easily set one up, or use these ideas to spark you into establishing a similar conservation effort, maybe on a local project which particularly interests you. These can sometimes be quite eccentric – removing undergrowth from a neglected Victorian cemetery, for instance, or renovating an old cinema – but are almost always a great way of getting more activity into your life. The BTCV volunteers also do things like planting trees and hedges, and conservation volunteering often merges with gardening (see opposite)…

Dancing

You can't stay still when you're dancing, so you will inevitably be getting some exercise. That could be comparatively little, of course, if you just shuffle about a bit, but the aim is not to do that any more. You don't even have to dance with other people; bopping around the front room to Abba also counts. One good trick is to monitor track length with your music, and try to dance continuously and energetically for about 10–12 minutes; if you wish, start with one 3-minute track, then go to two, then go on further, and stop if you feel any sort of pain or are very badly out of breath.

Styles of dance really don't matter as long as you are moving your body around; just go for it. If you want to go a bit further in perfecting some sort of technique, find a class where you can learn something fun and fast like salsa. Flamenco is another form of dance where age and shape are no barrier. Get inspired by watching a DVD of Baz Luhrmann's great film, *Strictly Ballroom*.

Dog walking

If you already walk a dog then you may well feel you are getting enough walking into your daily routine. But do remember that gentle strolling does not bring the health benefits of purposeful walking at a brisk pace, so check out your dog-walking technique. It's probably the same as most people's – an amble interspersed with a bit of throwing and quite a lot of shouting. This may, of course, be fine for an elderly dog, but it won't help *you* that much. If your dog is up to it, increase the pace and range of your walk, extending its length. Go out when the weather is bad, and don't just slip round the corner and take shelter. Gradually increase the amount of effort involved in your walk, and both you and your dog will experience the benefits. Some people even like to run with their dogs. When it comes to the throwing aspect of a dog walk, get a long rubber throwing stick that increases the range of a thrown ball – not just good for the dog, but a great way of increasing your exercise as you will probably be using more energy yourself. Most dogs love this, so will want more, and more, and more. Just make sure that you are walking your dog in the best way, so that it's not just you exercising the dog, it's the dog exercising you.

If you haven't actually got a dog of your own, or if your pet isn't fit enough, then there are always dogs that need walkers. This could mean taking over some of the dog walking for an elderly or incapacitated neighbour, or it could mean volunteering as a dog walker with an animal charity or local shelter. If you know what you are doing, they will probably be glad of your help; if you don't know what you are doing, learn. The great thing about dogs is that they need their exercise. So do you, of course, but with a dog you really have no choice. And dog walking is, of course, a great form of exercise for the whole family.

Gardening

Before you dismiss this out of hand because you only have a window box, you don't actually need a garden yourself. Guerrilla gardening is another way of contributing to your local environment, while also reaping possible health benefits; check out this burgeoning movement (www.guerrillagardening.org). Although mostly based in urban areas, you are likely to find guerrilla gardening going on in small towns and villages too – just keep your ears open and express a vague interest, and the next thing you know you'll be standing on a traffic island in a high-visibility jacket planting petunias. Weeding and litter collection are other aspects of guerrilla gardening that are always necessary, and some guerrilla gardeners have gone on to benefit their lives, and their communities, in another way – they grow vegetables. This is becoming increasingly popular whether you are a guerrilla gardener or not; there are waiting lists for allotments and a developing 'landshare' scheme in the UK.

Many of those with gardens are beginning to grow their own food now, if they have not already done so, and working in the garden can be a great form of exercise. Plus you have something to show for it at the end of a session. It's not just a question of producing a harvest either (though note that children will usually eat even the greenest vegetable if they have grown it themselves), but of the different forms of activity involved. Digging is obvious, exercising your legs, arms and shoulders, but raking leaves is great for your upper arms, as is mowing the lawn, and even weeding can be useful. Simply moving about in the open air is good for you. It's impossible to garden from a chair, so you are at least standing up and doing something.

Walking

It's so easy to add a little bit of walking into every day, and this is probably, therefore, the most painless way of upping your activity level. It's great, it's free, it doesn't require you to shell out for any club membership or expensive equipment and doesn't exclude any group in society, from the oldest to the youngest. You can walk anywhere, you don't have to live in the countryside; you don't even have to buy proper walking boots to simply get off the bus or tube one stop earlier and walk from there to your office – and adding 30 minutes walking to your daily routine is as simple as that. But don't amble gently along; that won't have the desired effect. You can encourage yourself to go faster by swinging your arms; don't let them come up too high or you'll overbalance (as well as look completely ridiculous on the way into work).

Walking has many other great things going for it; the enormous Nurses' Health Study, for instance, found that women who walked briskly for at least three hours in total each week had the same level of protection against heart disease as those who took a 90-minute exercise class – a 30–40 per cent lower risk. Research also showed an even greater reduction in the chance of having a stroke. In another study, women walkers had a much reduced risk of developing gallstones. Walkers in general are also less likely to get colds, coughs and sneezes, and another study even found that walking had the same effect on stress and tension as taking a tranquilliser. It doesn't put the same strain on the body as doing a more high-impact activity, and it has even been shown to help those who already suffer from pain, especially back pain; it can help to build bone density too. Finally, one recent study involving people with type 2 diabetes has shown that walking improved their bodies' ability to control blood sugar and reduced the effects of their diabetes. That's a fairly convincing selection of benefits for almost no drawbacks.

There are some, though … you can get wet and may be cold, so use lightweight waterproof outerwear and a fleece to keep you warm; a hat makes all the difference. One thing you may notice if you walk a lot on hard surfaces is that you get sore shins, resulting from inflammation of the muscle at the front of the shin, but you can help by doing a simple exercise. The fitness writer Joanna Hall recommends lying on your back with your feet flat on the floor, then lifting your toes towards your shins while your heels stay on the floor. Hold this for 10 seconds and release; repeat eight or ten times, and do so most days of the week.

Walking more can quickly become addictive, and you will probably want to add more than the extended-commute option. In the UK a good place to start investigating is the Ramblers Association (www.ramblers.org.uk), as they have many ideas and plans, and they are not only concerned with walking in the countryside; their 'Get Walking' scheme is based in towns and cities. Having said that, walking in rural areas is a wonderful way of spending your time, and one which can bring increased health benefits as the terrain you walk through is much more varied; hills, for instance, can increase the effort needed.

Then there are the various specialist types of walking – power walking, Nordic walking, and other variations on a theme (and before you dismiss Nordic walking as only being suitable for the very elderly – you use two sticks – research has shown that it burns 25 per cent more calories than walking normally at the same speed). If you get into walking more, you may wish to investigate these; they can be useful. And of course there are plenty of events to motivate walkers, such as the

Walking shoes and boots

As with other activities, if your feet hurt everything hurts – and when you are setting out on a walk that can wreck your whole day. Shoes and boots designed specifically for walking will have padding in the right places and provide stability for your ankles. It is best to buy them from a specialist outdoor shop rather than a general sports retailer, but that doesn't mean you have to spend enormous amounts of money (you can if you wish, of course!).

If you have decided to invest in a pair of walking boots, then always wear proper walking socks to try them on (and buy some of those, too, if you don't have any). While your new boots should fit with the socks on, they can make it hard to tell if the boots are too tight, so try them on without socks as well – just to check that your toes don't reach the front, that the boots aren't tight across the foot and that your ankle is snug but not uncomfortable. Then you need to put the socks back on and walk around the shop in the boots. If you can feel movement between your foot and the boot, you'll get blisters when wearing them, so make sure your heel isn't lifting up and there's no feeling of looseness. It should be possible for you to stand on a sloped board in a specialist shop, to see if your feet slide down and feel pinched; if they do, go up a size. Good retailers will do another check, but you can do it yourself. Unlace the boots completely and wriggle your feet forwards as far as you can, so your toes are touching the front. You should be able to slide your finger inside the boot at the back of the heel with 'a little friction'. Too easy, and they're too big; impossible or difficult, and they're too small.

sponsored mass walks undertaken for charity like the UK's MoonWalk for breast cancer awareness.

If you think you already do quite a bit of walking and don't really need to do any more, then check it out by wearing a pedometer. The best thing to do, like assessing your food intake at the start, is to wear it for a few days and look at the overall pattern (so include a Saturday or Sunday rather than just the weekdays). Make sure your pedometer is a good one, though, as many are unreliable. The chances are that you will be surprised by how little walking you actually do; a lot of people do less than 5,000 steps per day, which would really class them as sedentary, and the average is only 6,000. Again, think sustainable and try and up your step count gradually, increasing it by about 5–10 per cent week on week, and it will soon become automatic. Aim to get to 10,000 steps per day, or even more.

These are just a few possibilities, but there are many more out there, so spend some time on finding something that you will enjoy. It's obvious, but the more you enjoy it, the more you will want to carry on doing it. And don't confine yourself to one activity, either. There's so much to do.

8 Shortcuts to success

One of the great things about trying to lose weight is that many people have been there before. They've got to where you want to be, and they've picked up lots of useful ideas in the process. Anyone who has tried a support group to help their weight-loss efforts will have experienced the information exchange which goes on. Sometimes it may not be relevant to you (and the best-known support groups are owned by the food industry, so you may need to be open-minded, even sceptical, about some recommendations), but it can be extremely useful, especially when it is more informal and comes from fellow dieters. Not all of us, though, have access to a support group or would want to use one if we had, so here are some reliable tips, hints, shortcuts and words of encouragement which can help in the quest to lose weight.

Some of these are common sense and may seem obvious to you and some reiterate points made in the rest of the book. Where this happens, they are simply here to re-emphasise an important point that you might have missed the first time round. Use them as snippets – triggers that you can remember easily, and which can be used to help you on your way. For ease, they are grouped into broad categories.

How to eat

You might think this was straightforward and obvious, but there are actually many tips that you can use which will help you in your quest to lose weight, whether it's buying food in the first place, preparing it or actually sitting down and eating it.

Shopping for food

We've all been there – standing in the queue at the till, looking at the trolley and spotting the crisps, cheesecake or chocolate that has somehow managed to leap down from the supermarket shelf without any assistance from us … So be organised and make a list based on what you intend to cook, and only buy things that are on the list. Don't allow yourself to wander around a shop or supermarket in a random way, as temptation is likely to strike when faced with offers you can't resist. Just buy the things that are on your list, pay and go. Always avoid impulse food shopping (which can be expensive and wasteful as well as tempting), and shopping when you're hungry. Indulging in impulse and/or hungry shopping is a quick way to ensure that you'll snack on your purchases before they even hit your kitchen cupboards.

Avoid temptation

If you know there's something you really cannot resist, then don't keep it in your cupboards. It's common to persuade yourself that you are buying it for other people in the house, so don't fall into that trap, either. If you find yourself feeling tempted at particular times, try and work out why. Perhaps you're not eating enough of the foods that fill you up, or perhaps you've been cutting out the two healthy snacks a day which are recommended. And if you do find yourself thinking about food and contemplating a snack, focus your thinking on the very last meal you ate, being specific about it rather than general. There's some evidence that this might reduce your appetite; give it a try.

Read the small print

Labels on food can really help, especially at first, so check out pages 68–70 again. Remember not to pick 'low-fat' automatically, as low-fat products are often high in sugar to compensate; check the calories. A slogan like '70 per cent fat-free' means that a product still contains 30 per cent fat. And don't rely on portion size measurements or the GDA figures; go for those which are for 100g of product. That's particularly important if you are comparing brands, as then you're comparing like with like.

Anything described as 'giving you energy' is actually giving you calories, often in the form of sugar, and largely unadorned by other nutrients, too. These are usually marketed as 'sports' drinks or energy bars, but they're not as healthy as you might think at first glance. Easily absorbed glucose is what they provide, and your blood-sugar levels will be anything but steady afterwards.

Never assume, when it comes to slogans or brief descriptions on packaging; check the ingredients list and nutritional information panels and don't rely on words like 'healthy' as a guide. Apparently healthy options may not be quite so healthy in reality. When you are shopping and reading labels keep this mantra in mind: if you can't pick it, dig it or kill it, don't eat it.

Sit down

Never eat when you're standing up. That cuts out things like tasting too much while you're cooking, but it also eliminates chocolate bars at the bus stop. It has the virtue of being extremely easy to do – and to remember. This can also help any dietary amnesia that may be setting in too. It sounds silly, but the things you polish off while standing – whether it's leftovers, raw cake mix or nibbles at a bar – are the very things that are likely to be forgotten when you're trying to remember what you ate.

No television snacks

Whatever you do, don't eat while watching television. Evidence has shown that people who eat in front of a TV (or other screen) are liable to eat more than those who do not, and more than they would if they were not staring at the screen. It is likely to be down, at least in part, to the concentration factor. Concentrate on your food and enjoy it, and you are likely to find it more satisfying – and you will feel full for longer. There's another dangerous aspect to eating in front of a screen though, and that's that the food you do eat is more likely to be high in fat, salt or sugar. Even keeping a record can be distorted, as most people underestimate the amount they consume when they eat in this way.

Take it slow

Slowing down is good as it gives you a chance to really appreciate what you are eating; you'll find it more satisfying if you do so. If you find this hard at first make sure you are not being distracted, and try putting your fork down between mouthfuls. Chewing each mouthful thoroughly until it is a liquid before swallowing will aid the digestive process as well. Treating your food with respect is, ultimately, a way of respecting yourself.

Portion control

You can have almost limitless quantities of vegetables on your plate, providing they are not starchy (like potatoes) and that they have not been cooked or dressed with anything wildly high in calories. And the wider the variety the better, so that's everything from red peppers and aubergines to broccoli and mushrooms, carrots and courgettes, curly kale, white radish, asparagus ... there's so much choice, so experiment with unfamiliar vegetables and try cooking more ordinary ones in unfamiliar ways.

One way of almost painlessly reducing portions – especially if you are tempted to pile them high – is to use a smaller plate. Not a minute one, just one a little smaller than those you usually use. Plate sizes have also increased recently, just like glass sizes, so make sure you are not automatically using something which would have seemed enormous a few years ago.

Watch the overall balance of your diet and check that there isn't too much emphasis on things like rice, pasta, bread and potatoes, as well as the more high-fat items. Keep sliced bread in the freezer. If you do this, you can just toast a slice at a time and are much less likely to be tempted by quick snacks. If you bake your own bread, slice it before freezing.

Listen to your body

Various research projects have shown that we all have a powerful urge to clear our plates, or eat what we have been given, for whatever reason. Be aware of this and stop eating when you're ready to stop instead. You'll soon be able to adjust your portion size accordingly but you can always save or freeze leftovers.

Small glasses

If you regularly drink a glass of wine with your meal, a quick way to cut calories – and quantities – is to swap your existing wine glasses for slightly smaller ones. Research has shown that even if people intend to fill a large glass less, they still drink more than they would from a smaller glass. Also bear in mind that the average bottle of wine is stronger than it used to be.

Dietary amnesia is real

You can easily forget about things you eat or drink without really thinking about them – leftovers, a biscuit grabbed over a cup of tea – and one of the most common things to forget is drinks. If you're finding yourself stalling or gaining weight, check you aren't falling into this trap. A good way to beat the amnesia is to get into the habit of pausing for a count of ten before you eat or drink anything; that means you will really consider whatever it is and are likely to remember it even if you go ahead. Then at least you'll know the reason behind a stalled weight loss. If you're not keeping a written record, start doing so – but you can still fall into the amnesia trap.

Adapting recipes

If you find a recipe you fancy but think it would be impossible while you're trying to lose weight, take a look at the ingredients list. In a savoury dish the first thing to consider should be the oil or fat element:

does it really need *four* tablespoons of olive oil? Read though the instructions; the chances are that you can reduce that figure to a single tablespoon or even less. Sweet recipes often contain a lot of sugar which can be reduced, though don't expect too much from cakes.

You can also alter the proportions. A 'standard' fruit crumble, for instance, would have a thick layer of crumble on top of the fruit, made from fat, flour and sugar. You could reduce the quantities so the crumble was thinner, use oats instead of some of the flour, substitute wholemeal flour for white flour anyway, and knock back the amounts of sugar and butter in the overall reduction. Don't serve your crumble with custard or cream, but choose low-fat Greek yoghurt instead – it's every bit as good. Give it a go, and you'll soon see there's no reason to miss out on dishes like this.

Simple choices

As a shortcut, always use more of low-calorie, low-fat ingredients. If you are preparing stuffed peppers, for instance, make the stuffing more vegetables than rice; if you're making a pasta salad for your lunch, include much more tomato, cucumber and onion than pasta, and serve it on lettuce. If it's a traditional Sunday lunch that you're eating, have more plain vegetables than anything else, but go easy on the potatoes. Pad high-calorie choices with low-calorie ones, so have couscous with lots of vegetables rather than the other way round, and check out the muesli recipe on page 95, which uses grated apple.

Measure when you need to

Remember that heaped or rounded spoonfuls will contain more of whatever you are measuring than level spoon measures, and will also therefore contain more calories – maybe almost double. Most recipes mean 'level' when they list spoon measures in the ingredients. Weigh and measure high-calorie ingredients, at least at first – that would include oil and fat, cheese and many other dairy products, many meats such as bacon, sugar and starchy food like potatoes, pasta and rice.

Never, ever eat anything from the packet, and be careful about finishing off that little bit or indulging in excessive 'tasting' as you cook.

Keep an eye on your milk intake

If you are checking what you are doing by writing things down, you may suddenly realise that you are still drinking a lot of milk in tea and coffee. But measuring it can be a pain – are you really going to take spoon measures around with you? Instead measure some milk into a sealable container and use that milk, and only that milk, to add to your hot drinks during the course of a working day. If you have to put any more in the container, make a note of how much. At the end of the day, measure what's left (not forgetting to add any extra), and the difference is your consumption.

This figure can be quite surprising, and will probably prompt you into action, whether that's taking your drinks without milk or cutting down to skimmed milk. Full-fat milk has 66 calories for 100ml (most glasses hold 250–300ml), semi-skimmed has 46 and skimmed 32. The chances are that your milk drinking has added well over 100 calories per day, maybe double or treble that figure. You might drink more or less at the weekends, so do the same exercise on a day when you're not working.

Make your own ready meals

If you deliberately make more than you need – which is a great idea for convenience, providing you can trust yourself not to eat all of whatever you've cooked – or if you have leftovers, freeze them in individual freezer boxes. Soups, pasta sauces and casseroles are particularly good dishes for freezing and can be defrosted and reheated quickly when you need them.

Make sure you write a description of what's inside the container on the lid, however, along with the date, so it's not kept for too long. The general recommendation is that you should eat frozen fish dishes within four months, while meat ones can last up to a year.

What to eat

Avoid the diet bugbear, boredom, at all costs. The greater the variety of healthy food in your diet as a whole, the better for both your health and your weight loss.

Eat well

Don't rely on processed foods, whether that's ready meals or drinks which are supposed to keep you healthy. The best way of improving your health is to eat a balanced diet which comes from fresh, raw ingredients, and which has a marked bias towards fruit and vegetables and away from refined carbohydrates and food high in saturated fat. No 'functional' food, however good for you – and that's debatable – will ever replace a good overall diet.

Five a day

Really work to get to the target five-a-day portions of fruit or vegetables, because it is definitely worth it. Recent research has shown that if you get to five portions, you'll reduce your risk of having a stroke by 11 per cent. If you increase it further, that risk can go down by 26 per cent. Many vegetables and fruits are also comparatively low in calories and very low in fat, so you can fill up without damaging your weight-loss campaign.

Snacks

Don't forget to snack to keep your blood-sugar levels steady. Keep healthy snacks to hand, and as tempting as possible – crunchy slices of carrot, a juicy peach, a few black olives or a couple of slices of dried mango – and then you won't feel the draw of the sweet counter quite as much. Beware of superficially 'healthy' snacks in shops too – you would be much better off having an apple and a handful of nuts than you would buying a cereal bar. If you are without a healthy snack when you feel the need of an unhealthy one, resistance can be very difficult. Also, are you really hungry? You may just be thirsty (see below) or bored.

Don't reward yourself with 'naughty' food. Have a small handful of nuts instead; not only are they packed with nutrients, but several studies have also shown that they can curb the appetite. If you can't tolerate nuts, go for dried fruit, perhaps.

Choose soup

Studies have shown that soups really do fill you up for longer, so it is worth having soup several times a week. Make your own as you can control the ingredients (many commercial brands are high in salt and sugar, for example, even the ones which have a deliberately healthy, rural image). They are easy to cook and take no time, generally use the sort of ingredients that are best for you – vegetables and pulses – and retain a lot of nutrients. Adapting recipes is easy; you can cut back enormously on the fat used to pre-cook things like onions, or even eliminate it completely. Some soups use milk or cream; go for skimmed milk or stir some low-fat yoghurt into the cooling soup before serving instead.

Meat

Cut down on the amount of meat in casseroles, adding extra vegetables and pulses, and always remove as much fat as possible before using the meat anyway. Grill or dry-fry bacon and always blot excess fat with kitchen paper – put the cooked rashers on a piece of kitchen paper and press another sheet on top. Raw bacon freezes very well, and if you split a pack up into two-rasher portions before freezing, you can just defrost what you need.

Oils and fats

You don't have to use olive oil for everything; the taste is wrong or wasted in some dishes, such as strongly flavoured curries, and it is often more expensive. Nor do you have to pay a small fortune for rapeseed oil – it is often sold as plain vegetable oil, so check the labelling. There's also a common myth that margarine has fewer calories than butter, but it doesn't, unless it's a reduced-calorie brand of spread. Check these for the presence of trans fats (see page 58).

Dressings

If you like mayonnaise, then mix a spoonful of mayo with low-fat yoghurt to reduce the calories, rather than cutting out the mayonnaise you love completely. There are 'light' versions in the shops, but some leave a very odd after-taste, so you may prefer the yoghurt option.

Bottled dressings – whether that's just a simple French dressing or something more elaborate – are often very high in calories (as well as some ingredients you may not be able to identify when you read the label). They are also difficult to use with moderation, so don't run the risk. Use an oil-drizzler bottle, and buy another for balsamic vinegar, and then swirl them briefly over your salads instead.

Stay hydrated

Keep your intake of liquid up during the course of a day. Every cell in the body needs water to function, so make sure you are drinking plenty of it – six to eight glasses a day. You can count herbal tea, and ordinary tea or even some coffee according to certain commentators, but the majority of your intake should be plain water. You'll need more liquid when it's hot or when you've been exercising too. Steer clear of sweet soft drinks, fizzy or still.

When to eat – and when not to

Try to eat regularly throughout the day, and learn how to listen to your body – know when you're actually hungry as opposed to just bored or even just thirsty.

Eat regularly

During the day, don't go more than three or four hours without eating; have three meals a day and two healthy snacks. This is necessary to try and keep your blood-sugar levels as steady as possible, which will help your weight-loss effort. It is particularly important not to skip breakfast, and to make that breakfast a healthy one. If you miss meals you won't save calories in the long run – you'll soon become so ravenously hungry that you'll eat anything, and doubtless a lot of that anything; if you are really hungry, it's difficult to discriminate. At the same time, don't just eat because the clock tells you to; if you usually have lunch at 12.30, but you're fine and not at all hungry, wait a little – not *too* long, though.

Try a glass of water instead

Don't confuse thirst with hunger – dehydration can make you think you are hungry when what you actually need is something to drink, so make sure you have your equivalent of six to eight glasses of water a day. Keep a small bottle of mineral water by you during the working day, so it will always be to hand.

Eating out

Don't refuse to go out for meals when you're trying to lose weight – just keep your aim in mind.

Sensible precautions

Eating an apple before you go out is a good way of taking the edge off your appetite, and never be tempted to snack on bread or other alternatives while you look at the menu – ask for a glass of water to sip. Don't start drinking alcohol until you've had something to eat, either. There are ways of cutting consumption that are almost painless. You could determine that you would only have two courses, no matter how tempted you were, or you could anticipate temptation and agree to share a pudding. But don't order a dessert at the start – you will probably be full enough not to need one when the time comes.

Ask questions

If ingredients and cooking methods aren't obvious when you look at the menu, ask. Ask for what you want too; no dressings, no creamy sauces. Most waiters will be glad to supply the information, and if you are embarrassed just explain that you need to be careful about what you eat (well, you do).

Salads often come already dressed in restaurants; you can easily ask for your dressing on the side. You also need to be wary of sauces on vegetables, as well as on more obvious things like meat and fish, and you can ask for these to be served on the side as well. New potatoes are one of the many vegetables that are often served with butter; again, you can ask for this to be omitted.

Choose well

Go very easy on, or avoid, fried food, from fish and chips to egg-fried rice, unless you can control the amount of fat used – and you can't do that when you're eating out. Big cooked breakfasts are best done at home, and rarely!

Don't have the sugary chutneys in an Indian restaurant; instead stick to marinated sliced onion with a popadum and try a raita, made with yoghurt and vegetables – usually cucumber or onion – with a tandoori.

Puddings

You might think cheese and biscuits would be better for you than that pudding you would love, but bear in mind the high calorie content of cheese (and many biscuits, come to that). You might be better having that pudding without the cream than finishing your meal with a slab of

Stilton. Meringues can be a good option, but beware of the cream there too; water ices, granitas and sorbets are probably the best choices and are commonly available.

All you can eat ...

Buffets can be bad, as most people have a tendency to eat more than they need when presented with a variety of choices, so approach them with caution, whether they are in restaurants or at parties. The same reservation applies to salad bars; watch the high-calorie, high-fat choices, especially those slathered in dressings, and don't add more high-fat dressing, either.

Sandwiches

If you have no choice but to buy a sandwich at lunchtime, make sure you go for wholemeal or granary bread and a diet-friendly filling, and that means keeping it relatively plain but with lots of salad if you wish. Avoid the prepared mixes with mayo, so popular in most sandwich bars. You may find that calorie-counted ones are available, but check ingredients carefully. You can always turn your sandwich into a Scandinavian-style open sandwich and discard the top slice of bread. If you're buying coffee to go with your sandwich, then black is best. Some of the choices in coffee shops can be amazingly high in calories and fat, so wean yourself off them if you are an addict.

Fast food

Never supersize anything – even drinks. Be very wary of apparently healthy options, usually salads, in fast-food joints; they can be almost as high in fat and calories as the more obviously high-calorie choices like burgers. A standard portion of fries can have as many calories as an entire meal (and may be worth avoiding – it's hard to stop at just one chip). Another thing you can do, if you like an occasional burger, is to discard at least part of the bun, which many people do anyway.

Parties

These are dangerous territory, but are fortunately infrequent – for most of us. Again, think before you go and dance as much as you can; it's exercise *and* it keeps you away from the buffet and the beer.

Alcohol counts ...

It's all too easy to forget that the amount you drink has an impact on your diet. Not only are there calories in alcohol, but mixers can be high and make total calories shoot up. And beware of coming over all Rhett Butler after a few drinks ('Frankly, my dear, I don't give a damn'). Go easy. You can try matching alcohol and water as well, drink for drink, or 'baptise' your wine as the French sometimes do – add some water to your glass.

... and so do nibbles

Stand well away from any buffet table or bowls of nibbles at parties. That way you won't be able to help yourself so easily. And if you are tempted to nibble something, olives are a much better choice than most other bits. Avoid salted nuts, crisps, cheese straws, sandwiches, little quiches or pizza slices as much as possible.

Make it easy

Never, ever put yourself to an impossible test. Examples range from denying yourself a single chocolate when people are passing round a box, to sitting in front of your birthday cake saying, 'No, thanks, I'll have lettuce'. Set yourself up to succeed, not fail. That could mean suggesting an alternative to the birthday meal which doesn't involve food, or it could mean having a small slice of cake and sticking at a single one. Keep it real, and you keep it sustainable. It is also perfectly acceptable to have 'off' days, when you are not feeling completely well, perhaps, or are especially tired, but make sure they don't happen too often.

Exercise

It's particularly important that you increase your activity levels, and it doesn't have to be difficult.

Get fit

Exercise to get fit, not to get slim – if that's your only motivation, you will fail. Exercise is actually unlikely to provide weight-loss benefits as such, even when you're also eating healthily (you'd have to do a whole hour of intensive aerobics to burn the calorie equivalent of about half a Danish pastry, and you'd be liable to eat more than that to compensate for the energy used). It does seem, however, that exercise can help you maintain weight loss, probably because it helps you build muscle and maintaining muscle uses more energy than maintaining fat. And if you're fitter, you'll be healthier.

Move about

Sit in front of a screen less often, whether that's at home or work. Try and make sure that you move about more; walk to have a word with a colleague rather than sending them an email; get yourself a cup of tea. At home make sure you don't slump in front of the television for the whole evening; stand up and move around at least once every hour. Do little tasks that you've been putting off – wash up, take out the rubbish, do a little tidying. You could even do a few simple exercises during breaks.

Keep going

There will be times when exercising is hard: when it's raining too heavily for a walk or when the prospect of leaving a warm swimming pool with wet hair in cold weather can put you off. It is important that you stick at it, however, particularly if you are trying to maintain your weight, so try and deal with your objections realistically. Buy better wet-weather gear if you're getting soaked to the skin; wrap up warm and dry your hair before you leave the changing room. Sometimes these 'reasons' are really excuses.

Variety is the spice of exercise

In an ideal world, you would do some form of aerobic exercise (and that doesn't only mean sweaty studios and Lycra, it means swimming, dancing and brisk walking too) as well as resistance exercise – weight training is the classic example – and something which promotes flexibility, such as Pilates. However, the world is not ideal and exercise may be new to you anyway. Keep in mind the idea that while you should just do more, you should also think about doing more in different ways, and branch out when you feel like it. Swimming a couple of times a week and then going to a yoga class may suit you very well.

Involve others

Exercising with other people can help and that doesn't necessarily mean team games, which some people loathe. But going to a yoga class with a friend, aquarobics with a group of the girls, or taking up golf with your mates in the hope that one of you will turn out to be an undiscovered Tiger Woods – they can all be fun. It is also easy to involve the whole family in exercise, which can be very useful if you are worried about an overweight child. Kids are generally active, and will welcome the opportunity to hang off ropes on adventure days, cycle along safe routes or even simply do some skateboarding in the park. Many swimming pools have 'fun' sessions, which really can be hilarious, so do some investigating and get involved.

Walking tricks

Walking is easy and inexpensive to do, and brings real benefits. For most people, it's the simplest way of getting exercise. Explore your local area. If you live in a city begin by following a guided walk; you don't have to be a tourist to do one. It's interesting, though, that many of us walk much more when we are away from home on a city break, for instance, so play the city-break tourist closer to home. There are usually leaflets widely available at tourist information centres, but remember not to stroll idly around like a real tourist. There are branches of the Ramblers Association all over the UK, so make contact with your local one. Finally, many places have specialist walks – whether to spot birds, follow deserted railway tracks, hunt down archaeological remains or pick wild mushrooms – so check local press and noticeboards, whether you are at home or away.

If you really get into walking, think about walking holidays. These can range from the rough-and-ready (camping and carrying your own stuff) to the more sophisticated (you stay in hotels and the holiday company carry your stuff). The logical extension of this is the one-off experience, whether that means following some of the fabulous long trails in New Zealand or doing a sponsored trek along the Great Wall of China. You may seem a long way from it now, but that won't always be the case.

Staying on the straight and narrow

Everyone needs encouragement. Always remember that the healthy approach to weight loss doesn't even have to be straight, or narrow … Everyone wobbles sometimes. Just do your best to keep your balance.

Plan

Various studies have shown that people who plan in detail often succeed. Some have shown that those who make proper 'where, when and how' plans for a task are almost three times as likely to act on those plans as people who only have vague ideas about how they might reach their goal. Put the effort into determining how much you want to lose, how long you anticipate it taking and how you are going to get there, and you'll be more likely to succeed.

Fluctuations

Remember that your weight varies from time to time anyway, dieting or not (women will probably notice that their weight goes up just before a period, for example), and that the rate of loss can fluctuate too. Stalling is normal, so don't panic about it, and don't worry if your weight-loss pattern seems to be erratic. Keep an eye on the longer-term trend, instead. Losing weight is a real achievement, so don't blow it by giving up if you run into difficulties. Reread chapter 6 on problems you might encounter, and pat yourself on the back for having got to where you are anyway.

Monitoring

If you'd rather not weigh yourself during the process of losing weight, and can't find a particularly tight-fitting garment to go by, how about making a note of your measurements before you start and putting it in a safe place? Some dieters have used photographs in much the same way, and you could find it useful to get someone to take a picture of you looking your worst in every possible way and stick it on the fridge (but you don't have to) …

Write it down

Keep a food diary if you feel you are straying at all, and you may find it generally useful anyway. Make sure it's as accurate as it can be, and be objective when you look back at it.

Cravings and binges

Cravings and binges are a form of giving in to temptation, in a way, and certain situations may spark you off, so try and deal with them (and check out avoiding temptation, page 137). Yes, you may just have left too long a gap between eating your meals or snacks, but if that's not the case you could be bored or even eating for comfort. Some people eat when they are angry or depressed. The upside of situations like these is that it can be quite easy to redirect your energy by distracting yourself, so do something else that is unconnected to food – and once you have recognised the pattern, it can be easier to deal with it in the future. Then remind yourself that they happen to almost everyone at some point; you're not alone.

Keep the faith

Learn from any mistakes you make, rather than giving up. Think about them, try to work out what went wrong and why, then you are armed the next time the same problem – or a similar one – crops up.

Quick reference 1: Quick tips

Remember to:
- Eat regularly: three healthy meals a day, and two healthy snacks.
- Exercise more: whether that's formal exercise or increased all-round activity.
- Make it easy; no impossible challenges, no peculiar eating patterns.
- Cook as much as you can from fresh ingredients and don't rely on processed food (convenience foods, functional foods, ready meals) or junk.
- Keep tabs on the size of your portions; never have big piles of anything except vegetables (but not potatoes).
- Remember five portions a day of fruit and vegetables, more if possible, and don't drown them in sauces or eat them in high-calorie coatings like batter.
- Go for whole grains rather than refined-grain products.
- Watch the fat content of your food and avoid saturated fats as much as possible; try to cut trans fats out completely.
- Choose healthy snacks.
- Don't forget about drinks – alcohol, plus the milk and sugar in tea or coffee – and avoid sugary, sweet drinks.
- Concentrate on what you are eating, and don't eat in an absent-minded fashion.
- Monitoring and planning can help.
- Drink 6–8 glasses of water per day.

And hang on in there, because even small changes bring big benefits – and sustainability is the key.

Quick Reference 2: Resources

British Dietetic Association
5th Floor, Charles House,
148–9 Great Charles Street
Queensway
Birmingham, B3 3HT
Tel: 0121 200 8080
www.bda.uk.com

British Heart Foundation
14 Fitzhardinge Street
LondonW1H 6DH
Tel: 020 7935 0185
www.bhf.org.uk

British Nutrition Foundation
High Holborn House
52–4 High Holborn
London, WC1V 6RQ
Tel: 020 7404 6504
www.nutrition.org.uk

Eating Disorders Association
1 Prince of Wales Rd
Norwich, NR1 1DW
Tel: 0845 634 1414 (adult helpline),
0845 634 7650 (youth helpline)
www.edauk.com

The Vegetarian Society
Parkdale
Dunham Rd
Altrincham
Cheshire, WA14 4QG
Tel: 0161 925 2000
www.vegsoc.org

Women's Health Concern
PO Box 2126
Marlow
Bucks, SL7 2RY
Tel: 01628 478 473
www.womens-health-concern.org

Quick reference 3: Further reading

Brand Miller, J, Foster-Powell, K, and McMillan-Price, J *The Low GI Diet*, London: Hodder, 2004

Clarke, J *Bodyfoods for Busy People*, London: Quadrille, 2004

Clarke, J *Yummy*, London: Hodder Mobius, 2006

Denby, N, Baic, S, and Rinzler, CA *Nutrition for Dummies*, Chichester: John Wiley and Sons, 2005

Gallop, R *The GI Diet*, London: Virgin, 2004

Hall, J *The Exercise Bible*, London: Kyle Cathie, 2003

Hall, J *The Weight-Loss Bible*, London: Kyle Cathie, 2005

Hark, L, and Darwin, D *Nutrition for Life*, London: Dorling Kindersley, 2005

Lawrence, F *Eat Your Heart Out*, London: Penguin, 2008

Lawrence, F *Not on the Label*, London: Penguin, 2004

Orbach, S *Fat is a Feminist Issue*, London: Arrow, 1998

Paul, G *Perfect Detox*, London: Random House, 2009

Roberts, M *Fitness for Life*, London: Dorling Kindersley, 2002

Sacher, P *From Kid to Superkid*, London: Vermilion, 2005

Santon, K *Perfect Calorie Counting*, London: Random House, 2007

Ursell, A *L is for Label: How to read between the lines on food packaging*, London: Hay House, 2004

Ursell, A, et al *Vitamins and Minerals Handbook*, London: Dorling Kindersley, 2004

Webb, T *Workouts for Dummies*, Chichester: John Wiley and Sons, 1998

Willett, W *Eat, Drink and Be Healthy*, Cambridge, MA: The Free Press, 2001

Wills, J *The Food Bible*, London: Quadrille, 2006

Index